# YOUR ELDERLY PARENTS FAILING HEALTH.

## IS IT AGEING OR A TREATABLE CONDITION?

Third Edition

# Dr Peter Lipski
# Geriatrician

MB;BS MD (Syd Uni) FRACP FANZSGM

Your Elderly Parents Failing Health. Is It Ageing Or A Treatable Condition? Third Edition.

Copyright © 2022 Dr Peter Lipski.

Woy Woy Central Coast NSW 2256 Australia.

First Printing, 2019.

Second Printing, 2021.

ISBN-13: 978-0-6485047-4-0 (paperback)

ISBN-13: 978-0-6485047-5-7 (e-book)

A catalogue record for this work is available from the National Library of Australia

NATIONAL LIBRARY OF AUSTRALIA

Published by Dr Peter Lipski.

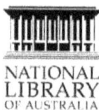

*The advice and strategies found within may not be suitable for every situation. This work is sold with the understanding that neither the author nor the publisher are held responsible for the results accrued from the advice in this book.*

# PREFACE

The 4 main reasons for writing this book include:

-extinguishing the huge myths and negative stereotypes about getting older,

-that normal ageing does not mean declining health,

-it's never too late to treat an older person,

-with good holistic medical care frail older people can have dramatic improvements in their health.

Old age will not kill you! Dr Lipski wants to improve the way the health care system is treating older people. This book has lifted the lid on misdiagnosis, malnutrition and other harmful medical myths.

Many families experience the frustration of watching their elderly relatives' health decline every day only to be told that it's just "old age" that causes dizziness, falls, confusion, malnutrition, and breathlessness and more. Families hear time again "what do you expect- he is 89 years old you know!" Too many older people end up in the overcrowded public hospital Emergency Department when this could be prevented by better medical care. How often do we see our elderly relatives or friends physically declining, slowing up, taking too many pills and struggling at home alone?

Many older people are denied proper medical care because their symptoms are commonly blamed inappropriately on "old age" rather than treatable medical conditions.

I have updated this third edition of my book to include more evidence-based medical facts versus fiction about the health of elderly people.

No one should ever blame old age for failing health!

*"Old age" is just a state of mind, it has no medical meaning!*

*"Old age" is something you should long for, not fear! I've always said that life begins at 90!*

*Never worry about "ageing", it's just a myth.*

*Don't ever let anyone blame illness on "old age"!*

*Remember, you are never too old for good medical care!*

*-Dr Peter Lipski 2022.*

# Contents

# INTRODUCTION

I wrote this book after seeing a huge gap in the public's knowledge about the health of elderly relatives, their families' great desire to learn more about how to help their elderly relative's failing health and general function, and what they can do to better support them in their older age.

One of the main goals of this book is to dispel the great myths, ageism and negative stereotypes about the elderly and growing old, what is normal, what is disease, and what is treatable.

As I will show you in this book, from my 40 years of medical experience and from evidence-based medicine, it is never too late to treat an older patient. There is usually something that Doctors can do to alleviate symptoms, potentially improve function and quality of life, and day to day function of even the very frail disabled elderly. Even for chronic irreversible conditions there is usually something we can do to reduce symptoms of chronic pain, breathlessness, agitation and distress. Even older people with dementia can still benefit from good medical care for acute and chronic medical problems. They can still undergo surgery when indicated for acute surgical problems and elective joint replacement surgery while they still have reasonable quality of life.

The greatest risk to the health of the elderly is ignorance, blaming "old age" for everything and presenting late to the Doctor. Many older people are in fact denied proper medical care because their symptoms are commonly blamed inappropriately on "old age" rather than treatable medical conditions.

Older people deserve the same active medical care that would be offered to younger patients taking into account their Advanced Care Plans and wishes. This book is not meant to be a textbook of Geriatric Medicine, but rather it highlights the very common issues and questions people always ask me about their elderly parents' health.

Geriatric Medicine has shown that with comprehensive care, accurate diagnoses, attention to detail, getting the simple things right, and treating reversible factors, there can be dramatic improvements in even the sickest and frailest older people. Whilst this book is not encouraging unrealistic or unreasonable expectations or benefit of medical care and treatment and not encouraging indiscriminate or unnecessary use of regulated health services, older people have the most to gain by comprehensive holistic medical care. This positive approach reduces hospital Emergency Department presentations of older people and acute hospital admissions by providing better medical care for the elderly. This also dramatically reduces health care costs for Governments and maintains quality of life for the elderly.

This book will affect everyone on the planet, as we all have either an elderly mother or father, brother or sister, uncle or aunt or other elderly relative or friend or neighbour. This book may improve access to appropriate treatment for so many more elderly who are otherwise fading and suffering with undiagnosed acute and chronic illness under the misconception of "old age". This book is also unique in that most of the topics discussed have been researched, presented at medical meetings and published by the author himself, evidence-based medicine.

There is one thing for sure, we are all getting older and living longer! At some stage in life we will all become "old"! If we get the right care and the right attitude to older age, then we will live a long, happy and fruitful life.

# "OLD AGE" – NO SUCH THING!

We are all living longer now. The average age reached now for men is 85 years and for women 87 years. However, I regularly see patients and relatives coming into my medical practice who are in their mid-90s. The average life expectancy of a person born today is 94 for an Australian female and 93 for an Australian male, and 50% are expected to live beyond these ages!

Many of them still look really well, are still driving, running their own households and giving advice and financial assistance to younger relatives.

A healthy older person-
- Has unlimited exercise tolerance.
- Can walk up hills and upstairs briskly.
- Does not fall.
- Does not get breathless.
- Does not get chest pain.
- Does not get confused.
- Does not slow down in movements to the point where it is affecting their day-to-day function.

Older patients can have spectacular improvements in their serious medical conditions because small interventions can make a huge difference to their health outcomes. Older people, like younger children, can get sick very quickly, but they can also improve very quickly with appropriate medical care. I call this simple "bread and butter" basic general medical care, focusing on reducing drugs and adverse drug reactions, treating organ specific disease including heart failure and infections, addressing low blood pressure, chronic pain, improving nutrition and mobility and their general function.

I have always said that life begins at 90 and that we shouldn't fear growing old!

Unfortunately there is an endemic, rigid, systemic, inflexible, irremovable belief in society that old age is associated with disease, disability and suffering. I was even taught this negative perception about the elderly when I was in primary school. Childrens' books illustrating older people greater than 65 years were showing older people as flexed over in posture with a walking stick (this may mean that they have neurological impairment with Parkinson's disease), they had lines around their hands suggesting tremor which is a neurological disease not normal ageing, and they were painted in a pale colour to suggest anaemia which is a disease. The message that came from these negative illustrations was that old age means disease, suffering and disability. These perceptions unfortunately persist today. I see this negative attitude in my daily geriatric medical practice. Patients and their younger relatives are equally surprised when I demonstrate the normal walking pattern, speed and balance of a 90 year old which is a very brisk and steady gait. Patients and relatives are also surprised by the following:

- That memory and brain function do not significantly deteriorate with age to the point they cause impairments in day-to-day function.
- Falls, confusion, incontinence and chronic pain are not a normal part of growing old.

Older people should be able to function just as effectively as a younger person. Daughters are the usual traditional carers of their elderly parents. They frequently attend consultations with me. The first thing that they say to me when I question their mother's general function is that "you know my mother is 80 Doctor" or "my mother is not bad for her age".

These comments again highlight the negative stereotypes and attitudes towards the elderly. The patient's daughter wouldn't say that their 21 year old daughter is "not bad" for her age, yet they say this about their elderly parents.

Relatives of elderly patients frequently become protective and say things like "my father has had a hard life you know", to try and compensate for their physical and cognitive decline. So statements like "he is 90 you know Doctor", "he has had a hard life" and "he is not too bad for his age" are all signs of the ignorance about what is normal vs disease in the elderly and that society in general has a very low expectation of health care for older patients. When I hear these comments it usually means that there is something wrong with the parents!

The "compression of morbidity" in the elderly, means that most diseases now are being pushed out to the latter years of life due to better nutrition and primary care through General Practitioners in earlier life up until the age of 65 years. Over 80% of all illness, disability and medical care are concentrated in the years after the age of 65 years.

Only 30% of over 85 year olds are dependent on others for day-to-day living. At least 70% of over 80 year olds are therefore completely independent in day-to-day living, giving advice and support to the younger people.

These days elderly patients in their 90's are having major surgery, aortic valve replacement, heart surgery and hip and knee replacement surgery with success. The oldest patient that I have had with hip replacement surgery was 100 years of age! The surgery was successful and he went home. He was still independent at home with some support.

Older people can have spectacular improvements in many chronic conditions with simple medical treatment including-

- Heart failure -with better treatment results in improved quality of life and less frequent hospital Emergency Department presentations.
- High blood pressure (hypertension) which results in dramatic lowering of risk of stroke and heart attack in the elderly, which can be very disabling.
- Osteoporosis and fracture risk reduction- for every 9 older people treated, one fracture is prevented- a very powerful treatment.
- Holistic general medical care and rehab focusing on multiple medical problems, improving mobility.
- Treating delirium and its underlying causes can produce spectacular improvements in confusion and mobility.
- Treating postural dizziness, adverse drug reactions and other causes for falls can dramatically reduce falls risk.
- Managing the behavioural complications of dementia with good medical care, reducing adverse drug reactions, and carefully using medications to treat agitation.
- Appropriate pain management can have spectacular improvements in general function and quality of life.
- Diagnosing and managing the cause of breathlessness can lead to improved comfort and exercise tolerance.

## COMMON LIES AND NEGATIVE MYTHS ABOUT OLDER PEOPLE

These false statements are so common throughout society, believed by most, yet totally untrue and promote the negative attitudes to ageing and older people. They confirm the harmful beliefs in society that it is normal to be impaired, confused and unwell from old age alone. These myths commonly lead to neglect of older people's health, and deny them proper medical care when they need it!

- Your memory worsens as you get older.
- Memory loss is a normal part of ageing.
- You get more confused as you get older.
- Your thinking and memory slows up in old age.
- Everyone gets more forgetful as they grow older.
- Confusion is a normal part of getting older.
- His memory is not bad for his age!
- She is pretty good for her age!
- He is forgetful because he is 85 years old you know!
- Everyone's memory gets worse with old age.
- What do you expect for a 90 year old.
- I hope that I am as good as that at 90 years.
- She has had a hard life, so I expect her memory to be worse now.
- She is not bad for her age.
- He has slowed up a lot but he is 92 you know!
- She keeps on falling but it's just her old age.
- I expect her to slow down and get more wobbly at her age. What do you expect!
- Everyone gets unsteady in old age.
- She is incontinent but she is 82 you know.
- You eat less as you get older.
- You don't need as much food in older age.

- He is pretty good for 90.
- She is breathless but she is 92.
- What do you expect for an 86 year old?
- Aches and pains are a normal part of growing old.
- He can't manage at home alone but he is 89.
- I wouldn't expect that he can do the things he could do when he was younger.
- It's just old age.

These terrible lies about older people put their health and life at risk because they end up being neglected by families who are in denial, but believe in these negative myths. Then the older person is just fobbed off and ignored when good holistic general medical care may help them and in many cases produce spectacular improvements in their health.

Many daughters and sons commonly tell me "my mother is 89 years old you know" when they come to see me in my private consulting rooms, when I only see older people. I study their medical file in great detail before I see them, so I obviously know how old they are! This statement about their age is just to let me know that their family expect them to be unwell or disabled in old age and it's ok to be unwell at their age. NO it is NOT!

## SUCCESSFUL AND INFLUENTIAL PEOPLE OVER 80 YEARS OF AGE

There are many very productive and highly successful people in the world over 80 years of age! Society tends to ignore and under value older people in general. Such older successful people who still made a major contribution to society when over 80 years of age include for example:
- Rupert Murdoch- Media

- Alan Greenspan- Chairman of USA Federal Reserve
- Henry Kissinger- Diplomat
- Robert Redford- Actor and Director
- Sonny Rollins- Jazz Saxophonist
- Sidney Poitier- Actor and Director
- Gene Hackman- Actor
- Chuck Berry- Rock and Roll Musician
- Chuck Yeager- Air Force Pilot
- Jimmy Carter- USA President
- Clint Eastwood- Actor and Director
- Tony Bennett- Singer
- Doris Day- Actress
- Larry King- Talk Show Host
- George HW Bush- USA President
- Buzz Aldrin – Astronaut
- Willie Nelson- Singer
- Irving Berlin- Composer
- Richard Strauss- Composer
- Clark Terry- Jazz Musician
- Richie Benaud- Cricket
- Reg Grundy- TV
- John Howard- Australian Prime Minister
- Norman Lindsay- Artist
- Bob Hawke- Australian Prime Minister
- Harry Triguboff- Manager of Meriton
- Frank Lowy- Businessman
- Elizabeth II- Queen of United Kingdom
- Winston Churchill- UK Prime Minister
- Sir Anthony Hopkins- Actor
- Julie Andrews- Actress
- Dame Judi Dench- Actress

So old age alone does not stop anyone from being active, productive and successfully contributing to society!

# PRESENTING LATE TO THE DOCTOR OR HOSPITAL

Unfortunately many older patients get to the hospital or Doctor very late in the course of their acute or chronic disease process. This is again because of the negative ageism and stereotypes of elderly relatives. Families expect that part of ageing is getting worsening back pain or knee pain, becoming more breathless, getting dizzy, having falls, becoming incontinent, getting more confused, slowing up and not managing at home. This could not be further from the truth.

If someone's 21 year old son was suddenly confused, incontinent, falling, in severe pain and becoming dizzy and could not manage at home, they would be taken straight to the hospital Emergency Department. Not so for many older patients. By presenting late to a hospital or Doctor, the chances of having more complications and having a worse outcome prevail, rather than coming early with new symptoms to get the best medical outcome for elderly patients.

## THE THIN RED LINE

Whilst I have always said that a person is never too old for medical treatment, there may come a time when they have been neglected for so long because "old age" was blamed for their physical or mental decline that they collapse with multiple medical issues and end up in the public hospital Emergency Department in a crisis. Due to accumulation of untreated multiple chronic serious medical issues including malnutrition, adverse drug reactions, deteriorating walking and balance and worsening confusion, they may actually cross what I call the "Thin Red Line", the point of no return when they develop serious life-threatening complications such as severe infections because of their malnutrition and immune suppression, and either succumb to their multiple medical problems or end up in a nursing home due to neglect and simple failure to get early appropriate treatment that could have kept them at home.

We must prevent the frailer older person from crossing that "Thin Red Line", to the point of no return.

## I DON'T WANT TO UPSET MUM

Dealing with elderly, frail parents who are unwell with memory impairment can be a major challenge. This is even worse when they lose their insight into their physical, cognitive impairments and care needs. Many families are unwilling to confront their frail elderly parents to try and get them some more help, to try and get them into hospital for appropriate care or to get them into appropriate Residential Aged Care. Many families are obsessed with not upsetting their elderly parents by just not dealing with their problems managing at home even when their elderly parents are starving, falling, getting more confused, drinking excess alcohol, forgetting to take their pills and self-neglecting at home. This lack of action usually results in a crisis, crossing the "Thin Red Line" and ending up in the public Hospital Emergency Department. The reasons why sons and daughters are reluctant to confront their frail, elderly parents or get them further assistance include:

- Confronting their parents to try and make them see reason will threaten their relationship.
- Unresolved, unreconciled relationship issues including unresolved guilt, conflict and lack of love in the relationship.
- Just want to keep Mum happy, no matter what.
- Watching their elderly mother or father fade and struggle at home because they simply just don't want to "upset them".
- Not taking executive action in getting the help that they need just because of the threat of anger and retribution from their elderly parents.
- Just unable to cope with mother being angry with them.
- In complete denial about their physical and cognitive decline, saying it is just "old age" when mother is actually quite unwell and could be treated successfully to resurrect her independence.

Many older people are petrified that they will end up in a nursing home if they go to hospital. With proper multi-disciplinary holistic medical care, most end up better, many with spectacular improvements in their overall condition and going home again with extra help if needed.

When our elderly parents become unwell, confused and lack insight into their care needs, then we really do have a duty of care to try and help them within reason. When our parents have lost the capacity to make rational decisions about their medical treatment, life affairs and place of living, Enduring Guardianship can be activated to make appropriate decisions to act on their behalf. Unfortunately if parents still have mental capacity to decide, and refuse help, then there is nothing we can do but wait for the "crisis" to occur.

A consultation with a Geriatrician may be of great benefit if the family can get them to the Doctor.

## I PROMISED NEVER TO PUT MUM IN A NURSING HOME

This is a fascinating statement as nearly 100% of sons and daughters who have promised this, almost guarantee that their mother will end up in a Nursing Home! It is a real paradox in life. The very reason that families promise this is because they can already see the writing on the wall and their elderly mother or father developing cognitive impairment and losing insight into their care needs. There is also a lot of associated family guilt and threats to the relationship with their elderly parents if the parents need permanent Residential Aged Care when they have significant dementia and they can no longer look after themselves.

I see many families inappropriately and desperately keeping their frail elderly mother at home alone for as long as possible with advanced dementia when their mother is clearly "beyond it" and cannot manage at home alone any longer even with outside help coming in. The family just want to keep Mother "happy" and avoid any arguments. They just can't cope with confronting mother about the reality of the difficult home situation and are petrified of her response and anger in refusing hospital admission, extra help at home or Nursing Home placement. This obsession about keeping mother at home commonly resides from family guilt when nursing home is mentioned but is clearly the safer option then. This situation commonly borders on elder abuse through elder neglect even though the family thinks they are helping and pleasing their mother. When their mother is unable to initiate and maintain their nutrition and hydration, forgetting to eat and drink, wandering, falling, poor hygiene with incontinence, unable to manage pills and socially isolated which makes dementia worse anyway, then the time has come for nursing home unless there are reversible and treatable conditions. We wouldn't lock a 3 year old child up all day at home alone, so why do families insist on keeping a frail very demented person at home alone when they are unsafe to be there anymore?

So watching mother or father "fade away" at home from self-neglect is not a sensible option. The challenges that then arise include-

- First of all family being able to recognise the physical and cognitive decline in mother and that she needs help. Many do not recognise this but simple blame the myth of "old age"! thus denying them proper medical care.
- Consent issues are so important here, so if mother has lost capacity to consent then Enduring Guardianship can be activated by the Geriatrician if mother has this to arrange extra help or hospital admission to diagnose the cause of the decline, find anything treatable and sort out the problems.
- If there is no Enduring Guardianship, then when does the family act to get help? It depends on the level of cognitive impairment, the degree of confusion and the severity of the physical and cognitive decline. Even if mother

has said in the past that she never wanted to leave home or go into hospital or nursing home, duty of care then overtakes this acting in her best interests when the overwhelming consequence of staying at home in self neglect and self-harm outweighs the person's wishes when they have lost capacity to consent. We just would not leave a frail confused older person at home incontinent, dehydrated, malnourished and falling irrespective of what they wanted in the past. Society has a minimum expected standard of ethical and moral duty of care here.

- Human rights, and self-determination for autonomy are just as important for the frail elderly but are extinguished in these critical emergency circumstances when medical duty of care overtakes impaired decision making in a very confused older person.
- Retained capacity to consent to life affairs, place of living and medical treatment means that we cannot go against the will of what our elderly parents want, even if it then means that they will continue to struggle alone at home. Then all we can do is to wait for the crisis, for them to cross the "Thin Red Line" and end up in the public hospital Emergency Department.
- Forcing older people to have care or treatment that they don't want when they can still consent is elder abuse.

Of course, a Geriatrician would always look for reversible, treatable factors which can help keep the older person supported at home if possible. The lack of insight into their care needs by elderly people who suffer dementia and the unwillingness of families to intervene results in usually a catastrophic outcome with a fall, delirium, malnutrition, self-neglect and a public hospital Emergency Department presentation when this could have been avoided by early appropriate intervention and care.

## AM I TOO OLD TO HAVE TREATMENT?

No, you are never too old for good medical care! There is something Doctors can do for all patients, even if it means adequate pain relief to reduce agitation and severe pain when physical function cannot be improved.

The reason that Geriatric Medicine is so successful is because there is attention to detail, getting the simple things right and a holistic overview of the whole patient, not just a specific organ approach.

Geriatricians specialise in major geriatric syndromes which include:
- Acute confusion/delirium, dementia, falls, walking and balance disorders, incontinence and adverse drug reactions.
- The frail elderly patient with multiple co-existing medical problems together including heart failure in the elderly, renal failure in the elderly, respiratory disease in the elderly, stroke in the elderly, Parkinson's disease in the elderly.
- Osteoporosis and fractures including vertebral fractures and non-operative fractures, fractured hips with medical management before and after surgery (peri-operative care) and chronic leg ulcers.
- Pre-operative medical assessments for fitness for surgery and post-operative care, with the focus on improving the patient's function and getting them home safely and effectively with help if needed.

Many Doctors are very challenged when facing long term disabled elderly patients who have multiple medical problems because their previous training has concentrated on organ specific disease, so their failure to recognise major geriatric syndromes such as delirium, dementia, walking and balance disorders, incontinence and malnutrition leads to deterioration of the patient's condition and avoidable Emergency Department hospital presentation and admission, resulting in increased health care costs and longer hospital stays.

A poor understanding of age-related changes in how drugs are handled in the body (pharmacokinetics and pharmacodynamics) leads to a much higher risk of adverse drug reactions in elderly patients causing enormous preventable suffering, hospital admissions and increased health care costs. A lack of expertise in these areas leads to inaccurate diagnoses. Lack of interest and expertise in the complex medical and functional needs of elderly patients leads to inappropriate transfer of elderly patients to poorly-equipped care settings and inappropriate referrals for nursing home placement when comprehensive multi-disciplinary geriatric care and rehabilitation would have made the patient functionally better and potentially able to allow them to return home to independent living, with or without supports.

## BLAMING OLD AGE DENIES OLDER PEOPLE PROPER MEDICAL CARE!

Just get a load of this! One of my 88 year old patients had a sudden onset of a very painful swollen right knee without a fall. He could barely walk. He went to see his Doctor who told him it was just "old age" and that his knee had worn out! The Doctor said that nothing could be done. The patient subsequently came to see me and told me that his right knee had worn out from old age! The first thing that I asked him was "how old is your other good knee?" In other words it is not "old age" that caused his knee pain, otherwise both knees would be bad. I subsequently diagnosed him with acute gouty arthritis of his right knee and with proper medical care cured his right knee pain and swelling to the point that he became pain free and could walk normally again! The moral of this story is never blame old age for any illness!

The end result of multiple medical problems in the elderly is usually falls and worsening mobility. This requires comprehensive holistic general medical assessments, focus on treating underlying medical problems, improving nutrition, reducing adverse drug reactions, and improving mobility. Yes, even the most frail elderly can have amazing improvements in their overall condition by this approach.

The most important preliminary step a Doctor can take is to get a very detailed collateral history from a spouse, relative or friend about the patient's pre-existing physical and mental function and how long has it been declining. A detailed functional, social and cognitive history from a reliable witness, followed by a thorough physical and cognitive examination, is the best starting point. From there an accurate diagnosis does require carefully planned and appropriate investigations.
I have previously written about these issues entitled "Optimum Care of the Elderly in an Acute General Hospital" (Medical Journal of Australia, 1996; V164:1:526). Ref 16.

# "THE WHITE PAPER"

I wrote this "White Paper" - A new direction for Geriatric Medical Services on the NSW Central Coast back in 2007 to highlight the need for a big change in the culture of the Australian health system to improve the care of the elderly in a more cost effective way for State and Federal Governments and to get better health outcomes. These principles also apply to other OECD countries.

The problem with the public hospital system is that we haven't changed the way we do things in the last 30 years.  We need to rethink the way we meet the challenges of our aged population and spread our resources between the acute hospital sector and the community. We have become far too focused on acute hospital care! Hospitals are focusing too heavily on "single organ" sub-specialty departments with a narrow clinical focus on one area of medicine rather than on holistic general medicine. We are waiting for the crises to occur rather than preventing them. We face a great challenge with the rapidly ageing population and its associated co-morbidities and disabilities confronting the acute public hospital system. The challenge is to provide safe, efficient and cost effective acute hospital and community care for our older patients.

## RAPIDLY AGEING WORLD POPULATION.

Western OECD countries are facing a massive tsunami of older people with their rapidly ageing populations. People are just living longer now with very long disease free periods until the latter years of life. The number and proportion of older

Australians is expected to continue to grow. By 2057 there will be nearly 9 million older people (over 65 years) in Australia (22% of the population); by 2097, 13 million people (25%) will be aged 65 and over and 1 in 5 older people will be aged 85 and over (20%).

More than 4250 centenarians (people aged 100 years or older) and super-centenarians (people aged 110 years or older) are currently living in Australia. Worldwide there were about 455,000 centenarians in 2009. That number is predicted to increase nine times to about 4.1 million by 2050.

The rapidly ageing population and increasing co-morbidities and chronic illnesses in old age will pose a huge challenge to hospitals and the medical system in the next 20 years. The elderly have a high risk of requiring acute hospital care, of rapid deconditioning and complications in the acute hospital system. In this older group any acute illness may cause preventable major geriatric syndromes including delirium, falls, loss of mobility leading to a prolonged, complex and costly acute hospital admission requiring prolonged rehabilitation and complex post-acute care. Ramping up multiple ambulances waiting outside Hospital Emergency Departments with frail older people with major Geriatric Syndromes is not a sensible or sustainable system!

## MAJOR GERIATRIC SYNDROMES

Over the next 20 years the major diseases and medical problems facing hospitals and General Practitioners given the ageing population will be:

- The rise in the prevalence of dementia and the associated behavioural and psychological complications including delirium and carer collapse.

- Adverse drug reactions in the elderly. I have previously published findings that 50% of geriatric patients older than 75 years presenting to the hospital Emergency Department are admitted to hospital as a direct result of major adverse drug reactions. The estimated cost per year for these 1000 geriatric acute medical admissions to just one hospital back in 2007 was estimated to be $10 million per year. These admissions are completely preventable and with appropriate community care, even at 50% reduction in these presentations would save just one hospital $5 million per year.

- Neurodegenerative and multifactorial gait and balance disorders contributing to falls and fractures.

- Osteoporosis contributing to both surgical and non-surgical fractures. The numbers of patients with osteoporosis is set to exponentially rise given that life expectancy is increasing. These osteoporotic fractures contribute enormously to health care costs by causing considerable morbidity and a prolonged length of acute hospital stay. There were 65,000 osteoporotic fractures requiring acute hospitalisation in 2007 in Australia. Osteoporosis related costs of care were $7.5 billion in 2007.

- Delirium in the elderly is:
  - common
  - life threatening

- commonly multi-factorial
- results in loss of independence
- high morbidity and mortality
- amounts for up to 50% of all hospital bed days
- increases health care costs by at least $2,500 per patient
- major contributor to inpatient falls in public hospitals
- major extra costs with rehabilitation and institutional care
- is potentially reversible in a multi-disciplinary care setting
- potential cost savings to hospitals by early screening for delirium risk factors and management was estimated at $2.5 million per year for 2,500 medical admissions in 2007 for just one hospital.

- Malnutrition in the elderly and its associated complications including falls, fractures, recurrent infections and a prolonged, more expensive and complicated hospital stay. For each $dollar spent on high quality nutritional care $10 is saved for the Health Care System with better health outcomes.

Given the high cost of acute hospital care and the limited hospital resources, a new model of care needs to be established for the increasing ageing population.

My 2007 prospective audit of Geriatric presentations to the hospital Emergency Department  showed that these patients were taking on average 6 medications, with the most common symptoms or presentations being:

1. Falls 30 %

2. Impaired mobility  33%
3. Delirium and confusion 29 %

## PUBLIC HOSPITAL EMERGENCY DEPARTMENTS

Current hospital Emergency Department (ED) practice routinely focuses on fractures or the injury sustained after a fall, while there is little systematic assessment of the underlying cause, functional consequences, and options for future care and falls prevention strategies. Frail older patients are commonly sent home without being "fully sorted".

Then if the Emergency Department (ED) Doctors try to admit these frail older patients under a "single organ team" when these type of patients have multiple complex medical problems that require multi-disciplinary holistic medical care, they simply do not fit into a "single tick box problem approach". So these single organ teams may be reluctant to accept the patient, resulting in multiple phone calls from ED in an attempt to find someone who will accept the patient. The bottom line is that the majority of patients in public hospitals are complex, frail and old! Yet the system is still trying to palm them off to single organ Doctors who do not address their multiple complex medical and psychosocial problems.

## NURSING HOME PATIENTS IN ED

Many nursing home patients are inappropriately sent to Public Hospital Emergency Departments after a fall or with other issues due to lack of medical care in the nursing home. Many frail older nursing home patients with advanced dementia are being sent into ED for brain CAT scans after a fall even though they are not suitable candidates for any surgical intervention even if they had a bleed on the brain. Many of the ED presentations of nursing home patients are driven by families who demand acute hospital care and the threat of Medical Board complaints by families who appear to be directing medical treatment decisions.

The bottom line is that there should be much better medical care and after hours medical cover in nursing homes to deal with complex medical issues. My solution is that all Public Hospitals should be attached to local nursing homes and provide 24 hour on call rostered medical care with Junior and Senior Medical Staff doing regular rounds and providing on-site after hours medical reviews as needed.

The lack of medical care in nursing homes commonly leads to a medical crisis such as falls, delirium, and infections that could be prevented and managed successfully in the nursing home by early intervention. The worst outcome is a frail older nursing home patient lying on a trolley in ED for hours only to be sent back to the nursing home more confused. So why doesn't a Cardiologist or other Specialists rather than just Geriatricians visit nursing home patients? Better medical care in nursing homes would reduce the pressure on Public Hospital Emergency Departments and provide better outcomes for nursing home patients. This would also reduce health care costs for Governments. Home visits save health care dollars and prevent hospital admissions. Nursing Home staff need comprehensive training to understand and manage dementia and the complex multiple medical problems in the elderly. But, a good question is who is going to train them?

## WESTERN MEDICINE FAILING OLDER PATIENTS

Complex elderly patients with multiple co-morbidities including physical, psycho-social and cognitive impairments present a major challenge to public hospitals and usually result in a prolonged, expensive and complex hospital stay.

The usual current model of "single organ" specialised hospital care for patients, does not focus on functional impairment and early mobility. Prolonged bed rest of the older patient is commonly associated with significant functional decline even after the initial clinical problems have been treated. More than 50% of all frail older patients do not recover to their previous functional levels even after 12 months after hospital discharge, causing increased falls risk, higher risk of readmission to hospital and nursing home placement.

Hospitals are increasingly being run by non medical, non clinical people (Managers) making decisions about the medical care of the older patients. This puts the health care of older people at risk and is just unsafe to allow unqualified people to make decisions about and manage someone's medical treatment. Too much hospital bureaucracy focuses on ticking useless boxes like teaching staff how to use a fire extinguisher and washing hands rather than looking at the big picture of how to screen for delirium, falls risks, malnutrition, adverse drug reactions, drug to drug interactions, monitoring lying and standing blood pressure, actually weighing the patient, testing memory and cognition. Another useless tick box is how long the patient had to wait in ED for treatment when the whole system needs fixing anyway to prevent the long wait, and rather should focus on the outcome of ED treatment- did the older patient get better or end up returning back to ED with the same problem unsorted.

It is not cost effective to put the majority of health funding for the care of the elderly into the acute hospital-based system when the greatest need is in fact in the community. By failing to screen and address the needs of high risk Geriatric patients in the community, hospitals are setting themselves up for a "tidal wave" of complex, frail, Geriatric patients presenting to the Emergency Department who could otherwise have been safely and cost effectively managed in the community without the need for an acute hospital presentation.

The "private rooms approach" with the specialist physician sitting behind a large desk looking across at a frail older patient should not be the only approach. My retrospective audit of 140 home visits at Gosford over 6 months showed (mean age 81 years, mean Mini-Mental State Exam score of 17.7/30) 77% were seen at home, 13% in nursing homes and 8% in hostels, only 3 of these patients were admitted acutely to hospital through the Emergency Department, 5 were admitted to the hospital rehabilitation ward, the majority having medication changes, community medical investigations and more community services. The estimated number of hospital Emergency Department admissions prevented by home visits by just one Geriatrician was at least 100, with a 10 day length of stay at least, the cost saving to the hospital was $1 million every 6 months. The home visit consultations also had the added benefit of early identification and prevention of adverse drug reactions.

The traditional acute geriatric medicine model of hospital care is not sustainable. There are just not enough Geriatricians to look after all the older patients.

All Doctors should be doing comprehensive General Medicine!

## **PUBLIC HOSPITALS ARE AGED CARE FACILITIES**

Both Governments and the public can't recognise that the majority of inpatients in public and private hospitals are elderly. For a start, most young people don't end up in hospital with a chronic illness. Even cancers in younger patients are now usually managed with day only chemotherapy treatments. Geriatric medicine and the care of the elderly is not prioritised as the No. 1 core business of hospital and community based medicine. Geriatric medicine is still regarded as a "side issue" and something that needs minimal support, but not in the centre of the "engine room" of all public and private hospitals.

Management of complex geriatric patients with multiple co-morbidities and common geriatric syndromes such as confusion, falls, malnutrition and adverse drug reactions should be the number one top priority for the Health system.

## COST SAVINGS OF $32.5 MILLION EVERY YEAR FOR A NEW BETTER MODEL OF GERIATRIC CARE in 2007 for JUST 1 HOSPITAL

- $5 million for 50% reduction of adverse drug reactions

- $4.73 million per year for DRG (Australian Refined Diagnosis Related Groups) Casemix funding for the diagnosis of malnutrition in the elderly

- $10.6 million by reducing length of stay through improved nutritional support for the elderly (2,500 admissions per year)

- $4 million per year for reduced length of stay in a multidisciplinary Geriatric Ward environment

- $2.5 million for delirium screening and management per 1000 cases

- $1.4 million through domiciliary consultations and community care of the elderly - 140 hospital admissions prevented per year

- $1.8 million by 50% falls reduction through improved monitoring of standing blood pressure (30 fractured neck of femur per month)

- $2.5 million saved per year through better and more comprehensive Electronic Medical Record reducing length of stay (2,500 admissions)

My White Paper was endorsed in 2008 by the-
- Queensland State Minister for Health.
- South Australian State Minister for Ageing.
- Victorian State Minister for Health.
- West Australian State Minister for Seniors.
- Federal Minister for Ageing.
- NSW State Director-General of Health.

The cost savings per year for Governments for better health care for the elderly are
- Australia $3 billion.
- USA $40 billion.
- UK £4.5 billion.
- NZ $564 million.
- Canada $4.4 billion.

Unfortunately Governments are still ignoring my White Paper!

# FRAILTY IN THE ELDERLY

Only 30% of those older than 85 years of age are frail. Frailty is a medical syndrome characterised by neurological impairment, either dementia or slowing of walking and impaired balance, osteoporosis, malnutrition, cardiac and chronic lung disease. There are different definitions of frailty including older patients with progressive weight loss of more than 5% of their body weight in 12 months, reduced exercise tolerance, general muscle weakness and decreased hand grip strength, slowed walking speed and decreased physical activity.

Age-related frailty is nearly always associated with chronic illness and multiple diseases/co-morbidities and is not a part of normal ageing.

The common causes of frailty include heart failure, chronic lung disease with extra metabolic demands on the body, malnutrition, dementia, underlying cancer, chronic generalised arthritis and walking and balance disorders.

Frailty is therefore a common clinical syndrome in older adults which carries an increased risk of falls, injury, disability, hospital Emergency Department presentations and early death rate. These people have a decline in physiological reserve in the body, deteriorating function across multiple organ systems and are unable to cope with acute stressors on their body, resulting in decompensation, infection, falls, delirium and an acute hospital presentation.

Note that frailty can be completely reversed if the patient is comprehensively assessed in a multi-disciplinary approach and the underlying chronic conditions are appropriately treated and managed. It is therefore important not to neglect the frail elderly, but to offer them a comprehensive assessment and treatment plan because they may be fixable. Sending a frail older person to a nursing home will not fix their frailty!

Remember that frailty is not a normal part of ageing! That's why 70% of older people are not frail! Frailty indicates that the older person is very unwell. These frail older people need holistic medical care which could result in spectacular improvements in their overall condition with proper medical diagnoses and treatment of their multiple underlying medical conditions.

# SODs

SODs are single organ Doctors. They specialise in one area of medicine such as cardiology (heart Doctor), neurology (nervous system Doctor), respiratory (lung Doctor), renal (kidney Doctor), rheumatology (joint and bone Doctor), haematology (blood Doctor) and gastroenterology (liver and bowel Doctor).

Many of my elderly patients are very attached to their single organ Doctors. They feel confident saying that they need to see "my Cardiologist" or "my Neurologist". Whilst the medical care for that specific organ issue may be okay, single organ medicine does not meet the complex medical, psycho-social and functional needs of the frail elderly with multiple medical problems. Most frail older patients have multiple complex medical problems affecting their daily lives, not just one single organ problem. Many of my single organ Doctor sub-specialist colleagues agree that the best care is with holistic multi-disciplinary geriatric medical care with the Geriatrician.

## MEDICAL MERRY-GO-ROUND

Unfortunately many of the patients I see have been on what I call the "medical merry-go-round", seeing multiple single organ Doctors including the heart Doctor, the kidney Doctor, the lung Doctor, the blood Doctor, the bone Doctor, the joint Doctor and the brain Doctor, but then are still not "sorted", so the General Practitioner (Primary Care Physician) refers them to the Geriatrician for a comprehensive over-view to see if the Geriatrician can sort out all their problems in one sitting.

The "compartmentalisation" and "single organ approach" to complex elderly patients costs a lot more money, sometimes 1000% mark-up for State and Federal Governments to pay for rather than the individual and more successful care of a single Geriatrician in dealing with these complex elderly patients.

When I first trained as a Doctor in teaching hospitals, we were all encouraged to do comprehensive general medicine. In fact, to become a Physician it was mandatory that when we were examined on presenting a "long case", we focused on a comprehensive holistic approach looking at all the complex medical, psycho-social and functional aspects of the patient's condition/situation, and looking at the impact of their medical issues on their daily life affairs.

However, since my early medical training medicine has evolved from good general medical care to much more organ specific single organ Doctor approach which is much more expensive and does not meet the needs of the growing number of complex elderly patients.

## DO WE REALLY NEED MEDICAL SPECIALISTS?

The single organ (SOD) doctor approach does not work to produce the best health outcomes for complex frail older patients, nor is it cost effective. No one is taking control of the "whole patient's treatment", just individual doctors ordering their own tests and adding in more and more medications just increasing the risk for polypharmacy (too many pills prescribed) and adverse drug reactions. I see this approach so often both in hospital and community patients. For example, oh the patient is breathless-let's get the lung doctor, hang on- ankle swelling- let's get the heart doctor, kidney problems- the kidney doctor, low blood count- the blood doctor, arthritis- the arthritis doctor, leg weakness, the nerve doctor. This is poor medicine and does not serve the patient well. In addition, the cost mark-up for these multiple SOD consults is between 500% to 1000% per patient, yet they are still not sorted out!

OK, so let's look at just one example of single organ medicine. Is it reasonable for a Doctor specialising only in lungs to only look at the lungs and nothing else? The lungs happen to be connected to the heart, circulation and other body systems! So by saying to the patient "I only look at and deal with the lungs" is that good medicine? No it is NOT! A broad wide ranging holistic overview of the patient and their multiple medical problems and how they are affecting the patient's general daily function and quality of life is the best way to provide cost effective medical care and the best health outcomes!

A Geriatrician practising holistic general medicine with a focus on the physical, psychosocial impacts of the multiple medical issues on the patient's general function and quality of life could be a 1000% cheaper and produce much better health outcomes. Comprehensive Geriatric Assessment and multi-disciplinary medical care are proven to be more beneficial for frail older patients.

Let's have the debate- do we really need an Endocrinologist to manage diabetes? a Rheumatologist to manage arthritis, a Haematologist to manage anaemia? a Respiratory Physician to manage asthma, a Cardiologist to manage heart failure, when a general Physician or Geriatrician can do it all plus look and the functional outcome of the patient? We do not need to spend more on health or build more hospitals. By following the principles in my book and in my White Paper we can drastically cut health care costs both in the Public and Private systems, and have much better health outcomes by reducing preventable public hospital Emergency Department presentations, by holistic better general medical care of older patients at home. I have shown this in my research publications and medical practice at Brisbane Waters Private Hospital. We are far too heavily focused on acute hospital care rather than community preventative care which is more cost effective and prevents public hospital Emergency Department presentations.

Too much of hospital care now is driven by "tick-box" medicine whereby protocols are followed instead of looking at the big picture, lack of thinking about the patient holistically, and losing the skills of clinical excellence. Young Doctors in hospitals are being taught this compartmentalised medicine to the point where medical teams now can't manage basic general medical problems. For example, any kidney failure is referred straight to the kidney (Renal) Doctors, high serum calcium and high blood sugar are referred to Endocrine Doctors, heart failure straight to Cardiology Doctors, anaemia straight to Blood (Haematology) Doctors. So we are training a future generation of young Doctors who will be de-skilled and incapable of managing complex older patients and their multiple medical problems!

Public hospitals tend to simply "patch-up' the patients as quick as possible and get them out! They don't look at the "big picture", they don't look at the underlying multiple chronic medical problems and their impact on the older patient's general function and quality of life instead of taking the better holistic view of the patient which results in better health outcomes, less hospital re-admissions, and reduced health care costs. I have previously published a paper on this (ref 16) "Optimum Care of the Elderly in an Acute General Hospital". Medical Journal of Australia 1996; 164: 5-6.

# WARNING SIGNS OF DETERIORATING HEALTH IN THE ELDERLY

If we accept that there is no such thing as old age and don't blame it on any ill health, then this book has already won. This is the most important message from this book.

There is just no such symptom as suffering from "old age". So, when I hear those comments from relatives of elderly patients reinforcing their age and telling me-
- "well you know my mother is 90, Doctor" or
- "she is not so young now, Doctor" or
- "she has had a hard life, Doctor"

then I know that these relatives are covering up and trying to justify "age" as a cause for their elderly relative's symptoms which could be potentially treated or reversed.

First of all, let's look at this generally. If an older person can't manage at home this is a huge problem. This is usually caused by a physical or mental illness. It is no different to saying that your 25 year old daughter can't manage at home, although at a younger age it could very well be due to a psychiatric or medical illness. However, you would seek attention urgently for a young person, whereas we delay until the very end for an older person until there is a crisis and carer collapse.

So basically any symptoms which can impair an older person's day-to-day function should be investigated, appropriately treated and managed. This includes-
- deterioration in walking and balance.

- dizziness or falls.
- deteriorating memory or confusion.
- new onset of breathlessness.
- pain.
- weight loss.
- incontinence.
- swollen ankles.
- or any other symptoms that are affecting their day-to-day life.  You should never blame age on any of these symptoms.  They are always due to some underlying disease process.

# NOT MANAGING AT HOME ALONE

This is a warning sign that something is medically wrong with the older person. The commonest cause that I see of an elderly person not managing at home is due to unrecognised cognitive decline and dementia.

Unfortunately because most of the public and relatives of the elderly expect that cognitive decline in the elderly is a part of normal ageing, then they don't get worried about memory decline until there is a crisis. So the older person with confusion usually presents late in the course of their disease rather than early when they have the best option for improving their condition.

Other causes of not managing at home are:

- Undiagnosed or untreated medical conditions including breathlessness from heart failure or lung disease.
- Acute confusion (delirium).
- Acute infections.
- Adverse drug reactions.
- Neurological decline in walking and balance, causing recurrent falls or postural dizziness.
- Deteriorating nutrition with swallowing impairment and progressive weight loss.
- Depression.

All of these conditions can be treated and managed.

# MEMORY LOSS AND CONFUSION

The older person's memory does not deteriorate to the point that it affects their day-to-day function. Confusion, memory loss and dementia are not a normal part of older age. Whenever I hear a younger son or daughter say to me that their elderly parent's memory is "not bad for their age" I am immediately suspicious that they have an underlying significant cognitive impairment or dementia. You would not say about your teenage child or 22 year old son that their memory is "not bad for their age", yet we do this with our elderly parents.

## MINIMAL COGNITIVE IMPAIRMENT

The fact of the matter is that only up to 20% of people over the age of 80 have what is caused "Minimal or Mild Cognitive Impairment" with a mild short-term memory loss which is not progressive and does not affect their day-to-day life. However, about 10% per year of these mild cases can progress to Alzheimer's dementia. Those with multiple risk factors can progress by up to 20% per year to Alzheimer's dementia. The risk factors for progression include-

- Previous head injury.
- Excess alcohol intake.
- Smoking.
- Previous strokes.
- Underlying neuro-degenerative processes such as Parkinson's disease.
- Previous episodes of delirium or acute confusion with general anaesthetics for surgery.
- Abnormal brain CAT scan or MRI scan with significant white matter changes.
- Primitive reflexes on examination.

- Depression.
- Diabetes.
- Hypertension.
- Shrinkage of medial temporal lobe (memory centre) on brain CT scan.
- Low level of education.
- Playing contact sport such as boxing and Rugby League.
- Reduced verbal fluency and word generation (semantic fluency for words in one category such as animals or phonemic fluency for words starting with a letter).

A common response from families when asked how is their elderly parent's memory- "Well, you know that your memory gets worse and slows up as you get older, so it's not bad for her age". NO, NO, NO, NO, NO! Just plain wrong! Your memory does not decline or slow up as you get older.

Many families either do not recognise or deny the fact that their elderly parent's memory is declining and assume it is a normal part of ageing. Therefore, they do not take them to see their Doctor until they end up in a crisis, either not managing at home or ending up in the hospital Emergency Department with an acute confusional state on top of their progressive memory loss.

If a 90 year old has a normal memory we should say their memory is normal rather than "normal for their age". Impairment of mental function and a progressive short-term memory loss needs to be investigated to see if there are any reversible causes and to diagnose dementia and treat it appropriately.

# DEMENTIA/ALZHEIMER'S DISEASE

Dementia is a progressive neurodegenerative disease of the brain. It is incurable. It is not a part of normal ageing. Up to 10% of people over 70 years of age will develop dementia and up to 25% of people over the age of 80 years will develop Alzheimer's dementia. Dementia is the second leading cause of death of Australians contributing to 5.5% of all deaths in males and 10.5% of all deaths in females each year. The number of people with dementia in Australia is expected to increase to 590,000 by 2028 and 1,076,000 by 2058. Worldwide number was 50 million people in 2017. The number of people with dementia worldwide will double every 20 years, reaching 75 million in 2030 and 131 million in 2050.

Alzheimer's disease is the most common form of dementia. Relatives often get confused about the difference between dementia and Alzheimer's disease. Dementia is a general term to describe the syndrome of different forms of dementia. Alzheimer's disease is just one form of dementia. There are several other sub-types of dementia.

Alzheimer's dementia affects memory, thinking, behaviour and ability to manage your daily life activities. The typical features of Alzheimer's disease include a progressive short-term memory decline over several years. (If there is sudden onset of confusion, this is not dementia but delirium which is potentially a medical emergency and needs to be sorted out straight away.) As the disease progresses other symptoms develop including impairments of thinking, information processing, problem-solving and planning your day (executive function). Speed of information processing and thinking slows right down. It affects the ability to communicate, find the right words, express yourself and understand conversation (dysphasia).  It impairs the ability to focus and pay attention, particularly when the person is in a group conversation.  It can affect reasoning, judgement and also what we call visuospatial perception in space, getting lost in familiar environments even around the house, misplacing things, not understanding safe distance with driving. It affects coordination and planning of basic tasks such as cooking, even making a cup of tea or coffee (apraxia). Changes in behaviour, mood disturbances and psychiatric symptoms can develop including anger, irritability, verbal aggression, depression, hallucinations and paranoid delusions. One of the first signs of dementia may in fact be unexplained weight loss, decreased appetite and generally slowing up physically and mentally. Another typical early feature is being generally vague. Then the short term memory impairment starts to appear.

The hallmark of Alzheimer's disease is a slow, progressive decline in short-term memory-
- The person becomes  more forgetful.
- They forget days, dates, appointments and recent events.
- They can forget conversation a few hours later.
- They tend to repeat themselves several times over or ask the same questions.
- Losing train of thought and what they were going to say during conversation.
- Not able to follow conversation.
- They regularly misplace things around the house including their keys, wallet and purse.
- One of the first signs maybe loss of interest in things generally, and not doing their usual hobbies anymore.
- Loss of motivation- apathy, inertia.

- Sleeping more during the day.
- Slowing down mentally and physically.
- Deteriorating appetite, loss of interest in food, meals getting smaller and smaller.
- Unexplained weight loss.
- Personality change such as labile emotion, disinhibited social behaviour, lack of social graces, over- familiar with strangers
- Executive function impairments such as problem solving, new learning capacity, reasoning, information processing, planning the day's activities, everyday general tasks
- Repeating the same questions- "where are we going now?", "what are we doing next?" "what time is my appointment?"

As the cognitive decline worsens the memory loss can start to affect their daily life and routines. This includes:

- Difficulty remembering phone numbers, planning their day and forgetting to pay their bills.
- Difficulty completing normal routines at home including operating household appliances such as the microwave, dishwasher or washing machine.
- Dyspraxia -impaired co-ordination of simple tasks such as using the kettle, making a cup of tea and toast.
- Difficulty using the TV/DVD player, computer.
- Difficulty reading a book, magazine or newspaper or remembering what they have read.
- Difficulty following a TV programme
- As their dementia progresses they will have difficulties getting the right words out in conversation and understanding words, and have difficulty naming objects (dysphasia).
- Not recognising / remembering family members or familiar friends (agnosia).

- Management of their finances deteriorates and they either forget where they have put their money, withdrawing too much money from their account for what they need or giving money away particularly to strangers.
- Forgetting to pay bills
- Withdrawing from social activities.
- Changes in mood and personality, becoming either increasingly agitated and more aggressive or more subdued and withdrawn.
- Difficulty learning new things.
- Difficulty writing a card or letter to friends or a business letter.
- Forgetting to cook and eat.
- Forgetting how to cook meals.
- Missing meals.
- Leaving the taps or stove on.
- Forgetting to shower.
- Getting more agitated particularly in the afternoon.
- More argumentative.
- Refusing outside help when they are clearly not managing alone at home.
- Increasing suspicious paranoid behaviour against family.
- Forgetting to take pills/medications.
- Refusing to eat or having just tiny meals.
- Weight loss from poor appetite.
- Forgetting the name of their usual Doctor.
- Not remembering the name of and not knowing why they are seeing a new medical Specialist.

A common presentation of somebody with undiagnosed Alzheimer's dementia is that they can't cope alone at home any longer. This is not old age!

## MUM'S MEMORY GOT A LOT WORSE SOON AFTER DAD DIED

Families often report that when their Father died, they noticed soon after that Mother's short term memory and general confusion got a lot worse. Then they notice that Mother is not coping alone at home and just can't manage the house and daily life. It then becomes obvious that Mother had a pre-existing cognitive decline and early dementia when her husband was still alive, but he "covered up" and compensated for her by doing everything for her. Family did not recognise the cognitive decline until their Father died. Then they notice that Mother can't manage the finances or pay the bills, can't cook or shop and is struggling alone at home. This is a common scenario with unrecognised dementia where the partner compensates for the cognitive and functional decline, but the person decompensates in daily life soon after when their partner is no longer at home to prompt, support and remind her what to do. Then they end up in a crisis. This dementia should have been picked up well before by a routine health check and cognitive screening by the family Doctor!

## COGNITIVE FUNCTION IS ESSENTIAL FOR SAFE DRIVING

These are impaired in somebody with Alzheimer's dementia and they include:

- Speed of thinking/information processing.
- Reaction time/reflexes.
- Left/right orientation.
- Geographic orientation.
- Impulsivity and control of their emotions and reflexes.
- Visual vigilance/concentration.

- Not being easily distracted.
- Managing dual simultaneous stimuli.
- Sustained attention.
- Divided attention.
- Switching attention.
- Responding to visual stimuli.

These are the reasons why people with even mild, early Alzheimer's dementia cannot drive a car safely.

## EARLY DIAGNOSIS OF DEMENTIA

The reason for diagnosing dementia early is to manage the progressive cognitive decline, its impact on the day-to-day life of the patient and also its effect on family, friends and other relatives. Early diagnosis allows for an early medical management plan and drug treatment if possible, allows the person with dementia, their family and care givers to plan for future living arrangements and care options, to organise their financial affairs and make decisions relating to Power of Attorney and Enduring Guardianship.

Early diagnosis encourages the medical focus and assessment for-
- Minimising adverse drug reactions.
- Reviewing any drugs that may worsen the confusion.
- Comprehensive Geriatric Medical Assessment to minimise the impact of other co-morbidities (illnesses) the person may have as well.
- Swallowing disorders.
- Nutrition.
- Monitoring of standing BP as low BP can occur in dementia.
- Incontinence management.

- Walking and balance which can decline in dementia.
- Reducing falls risk.
- Management of any behavioural complications.
- Occupational Therapy assessment of the safety of the home environment.
- Community Services and extra help at home for the Carer.
- Safety ID bracelet or GPS watch for wanderers.
- Dementia Carer Support Group for Family and Carers.
- Respite care for Carer.

Alzheimer's disease develops in the brain years before symptoms develop. Accumulation of abnormal proteins such as beta-Amyloid which clump between brain nerve cells cause plaques and abnormal hyperphosphorylated Tau protein cause abnormal neurofibrillary tangles, both destroy brain nerve cells. Whilst these abnormal proteins can be measured using biomarkers and enhance the diagnosis of early Alzheimer's dementia, they are expensive and invasive, and still regarded as research tools so are not used routinely. These biomarkers include measuring Amyloid and Tau proteins in CSF (cerebrospinal fluid), blood tests for amyloid, amyloid brain PET scan, FDG PET brain scan looking for hypometabolism (reduced brain function). However the most important way to diagnose Alzheimer's dementia is with a detailed history from the patient, collateral history from family and friends about memory loss and general function, clinical exam and cognitive testing. Early signs of Alzheimer's dementia even before memory loss is evident include unexplained weight loss, slowing down physically and cognitively, and new anxiety and depression.

## WHY IS DEMENTIA DIAGNOSIS DELAYED IN THE ELDERLY

The simple reason is that many people including families and even some Doctors think that dementia and confusion are just "old age". How wrong can you get! A Doctor must always take the patient and family seriously when they are concerned about forgetfulness and memory loss. This should never be dismissed as "old age". The patient and family would be acutely aware of memory loss symptoms if they are concerned and report them. Again I say if a teenager was losing their memory or getting more confused then we would do something about it for sure and get help pretty quicky! I see many older people with very significant dementia who have been getting more confused for years with nothing done about it. They commonly come to me very late when their dementia is quite advanced. Unfortunately their families just suffer in silence.

Some of the reasons for late dementia presentation and what families say about it include:

-blaming "old age" for confusion and memory loss.

-just ignoring the problem.

-"my father has a lazy mind" -families in denial.

-families and Doctors saying "what do expect-he is 88 years old, it's just old age".

-"my mother has had a hard life".

-"my father has always had a bad memory".

-"my mother has always repeated the same conversation all of her life". (just an excuse to cover up for her cognitive decline).

-"he has good and bad days"-(family in denial).

-"other older people get confused", "it's normal for older people to be forgetful and repeat themselves!"- NO IT IS NOT! So families use this as an excuse to accept the memory loss as "normal".

-"if you compare my mother with others her age she is not too bad you know."
-"Mother refuses outside help and says that there is nothing wrong with her!"
-"my mother's memory is better than mine!"

Many families feel very threatened by the diagnosis of dementia in their elderly parents so make every excuse to avoid it. They don't want to face the consequences of having a mother or father with dementia, particularly if they live alone. Some family members even get very angry with the Doctor when dementia is diagnosed because they regard it as an insult or threat to their parents. They just can't see it so they just don't accept it.

The lack of insight into care needs when older parents have dementia is a common cause for crossing the "Thin Red Line" and ending up in crisis and into the public Hospital Emergency Department.

Old age must never be blamed for confusion, memory loss and dementia.

## WHY DIDN'T MUM'S DOCTOR DIAGNOSE HER DEMENTIA BEFORE?

This is a common but very worrying occurrence when the family Doctor or Specialist fails to recognise significant cognitive impairment, memory loss and dementia. This can lead to very poor outcomes if the patient develops an acute illness or is referred for surgery which commonly results in a post-operative delirium, post-operative cognitive decline and immobility. The delay in diagnosis of dementia results in denial of proper care for the patient, unnecessary carer stress and suffering for both the patient and the family. Common reasons for not diagnosing dementia include:

- Doctor saying that memory loss is just "normal old age" or it's just normal to be forgetful as you get older. This is so wrong, not evidence-based, ageist, and negligent. This is so inappropriate and lacks any science behind this statement- just a lame excuse not to bother helping the patient and the family!
- Doctor not bothering to formally screen for cognitive impairment with validated memory tests. Just talking to the patient generally and then saying that they seem "pretty good for their age" lacks any scientific validity. Many patients with cognitive impairment have excellent verbal and social skills to hide their significant cognitive impairments. Without formally testing them, dementia can be easily missed in the early stages.
- Specialist just not interested in the cognitive impairment. This is just a cop out for those not willing to sort out the patient properly!
- Specialist saying that's not my area of medicine? But it should be for all Specialists looking after older people!
- Doctors looking at just one thing only and not the whole patient.
- Doctors lacking the skills necessary to identify, diagnose and manage cognitive impairment and dementia.

## BEHAVIOURAL COMPLICATIONS OF DEMENTIA

Nearly half of the patients I see develop behavioural and psychological complications of dementia. These are very challenging behaviours that can cause massive carer stress and carer collapse, the common cause of the relative or family requesting permanent nursing home care as they can no longer manage.

If these behavioural issues are identified, diagnosed and managed early, then they have the potential to be treated and can respond to some drugs and non-drug strategies. These behavioural complications include verbal and physical aggression, wandering behaviours and getting lost, agitation, sexual disinhibition, depression, visual and auditory hallucinations and paranoid delusions accusing spouse, relatives or friends of stealing things from them or accusing their spouse of having an affair.

Other major behavioural problems include afternoon "sundowning" agitation where the dementia sufferer becomes more irritable, agitated and aggressive in the afternoon when they become tired. They become more confused and disorientated. They have insomnia, getting up constantly at night, wandering around the house. They can get day/night disorientation so they get dressed at midnight to go to work or demand breakfast at 1am. Urinary or faecal incontinence is a common complication of advanced dementia and difficulty finding the toilet with worsening personal hygiene.

For severe agitation and aggression there are medications available which can help control these distressing symptoms. These include cautious use of anti-psychotic medication, anti-depressants or other sedative medication in low dose. There is always the balance between the benefits of the medications in reducing the agitation, aggression and distress, allowing the patient to be managed at home vs drug side effects including drowsiness, postural dizziness and increased falls risk.

Most of the patients whom I see with advanced dementia and serious behavioural complications require drug treatment to manage their challenging behaviours and distress. This is almost always the case for those patients in nursing homes and Residential Aged Care, who already have had the expertise of nursing staff to try and develop routines and strategies to manage these behaviours without drugs and without success. Playing old movies, favourite music, looking at family photos and holding a doll just don't work for psychotic, paranoid and aggressive dementia patients. Lately there seems to be a big push for these non-drug behavioural strategies to control these difficult and frequently aggressive behaviours.

Governments are discouraging the first use of anti-psychotic medications, preferring these non-drug strategies which just do not work. The result is that the dementia patient suffers from ongoing untreated agitation and distress and well as causing severe carer stress and affecting the health of the carer.

Typical dementia behaviours that may require drug treatment include-
- Severe agitation
- Physical aggression
- Threatening behaviours
- Paranoid delusion
- Distressing hallucinations
- Acting out delusions such as wanting to call the Police for strangers in the house who are not there
- Night time restlessness and wanting to get dressed at 1am for work and leave home
- Afternoon irritability and aggression

- Accusing partner of having affairs and threatening them.

There can be tremendous relief for both the patient and carer with cautious drug treatment, monitoring carefully for side effects and regular reviews of progress. Such drug treatment can in fact prolong the ability of the carer to manage the dementia patient at home, delay nursing home admission and improve their quality of life.

## SWALLOWING DYSPRAXIA

They can develop impairment of swallowing coordination (swallowing dyspraxia) and have what is called a post swallow cough after liquids, so that when they are having water, juice, coffee or tea after every swallow or second swallow they start coughing because it is going down the wrong way. They can also cough after swallowing solid food. Therefore, they may benefit from a speech pathology assessment of their swallowing.

I generally recommend in these situations that the person be sitting upright and forward to reduce the risk of "silent aspiration" (food or fluid going down the wrong way into the lungs which will cause increased risk for chest infection and pneumonia, which is a common cause of death in these patients). They should have supervised meals where they swallow small amounts and if food is too difficult to swallow then it should be cut up finely with gravy to assist with swallowing. Sometimes the Speech Pathologist may recommend thickened fluids which may be easier for the patient with dementia and impaired swallowing to cope with and reduce the risk of it going down the wrong way. Unfortunately many patients hate thickened fluids, as there is nothing worse than having thickened tea or coffee. If it is more than Level 1 it could be as thick as honey and unpalatable. Then they are at risk of dehydration and kidney failure if they don't drink enough fluid.

## MEMORY DRUGS

There are memory drugs that may help slow down the memory decline in 1/3rd of patients. These are Acetyl Cholinesterase inhibitors, but 1/3rd of patients could get severe nausea and diarrhoea, in which case the drug needs to be ceased. These drugs do not cure the condition, but may slow the down the decline a little, or even make them a little brighter, more interactive, less agitated. Of course it is also important to reduce, withdraw and stop drugs that are contributing to worsening confusion such as sleeping pills, other sedative medications, anti-depressants, narcotic analgesics and other pain killers, and Parkinson's disease meds and change to alternatives where possible.


Patients with dementia tend to become "hypercatabolic". In other words, their metabolic rate increases and they begin to lose weight. This is despite eating adequate amounts of calories and protein. Progressive weight loss is a common early sign of Alzheimer's dementia and it does not have a good prognosis.

There are many patients with Alzheimer's dementia around the world. They can be successfully managed at home if appropriately diagnosed and treated and family supported. Most of my patients with Alzheimer's dementia can still be successfully supported at home with their family and loved ones after they have had a multi-disciplinary assessment, holistic care, careful assessment of their medications, reducing adverse drug reactions and focusing on their other medical conditions and physical function including their nutrition, their swallowing, their balance and mobility.

Dementia may be part of a general neuro-degenerative decline. I commonly see patients with dementia who also have gait and balance disorders and frequent falls. Dementia can cause gait dyspraxia or incoordinated balance and walking in that the dementia sufferer does not know where to put their feet and how to plan their walking. They generally slow up, can shuffle and look like Parkinson's disease, but it is not.

In order to maximise physical function and support a patient with dementia at home, they must have accurate diagnoses and management of their other chronic medical conditions.

A common, frequent and recognised complication of dementia is autonomic neuropathy causing postural hypotension. This means that there is a degeneration in the brain stem at the bottom of the brain which controls blood pressure and so the blood pressure drops when they stand. This commonly worsens their confusion and increases the falls risk. This can be managed with improving their oral hydration and using medications to elevate their blood pressure including Fludrocortisone if needed.

I always give the carers of my patients with Alzheimer's dementia a delirium brochure which highlights to the family what is sudden confusion/acute confusion and delirium, which usually requires urgent medical attention. This is different from the slow progressive decline of dementia. Delirium usually requires acute hospital care to find the cause and if the cause of the delirium is accurately diagnosed and managed, there is a reasonable chance of success for the patient with dementia returning to their usual level of function.

## AVOID GENERAL ANAESTHETICS

Patients with dementia should generally avoid general anaesthetics and surgery unless absolutely necessary due to the risks of post-operative delirium and further progressive post-operative cognitive decline. However, this is not to say that people with Alzheimer's dementia cannot have surgery, they can! I have had many patients over the years with Alzheimer's dementia who required abdominal surgery for bowel obstruction, hip fracture following falls and even elective knee replacement surgery or hip replacement surgery for severe weight-bearing pain in those joints with successful outcomes. These patients can have sophisticated regional anaesthetics with sedation, local nerve blocks and spinal blocks to avoid the complications of full anaesthetics.
If the patient has a reasonable quality of life and function at home, despite the dementia, the label of dementia does not mean they cannot have further active medical care if indicated.

While there is a risk of worsening their memory loss and confusion with surgery, by appropriately selecting patients who would benefit from a hip or knee replacement to maintain their mobility and reduce their pain and suffering, then this is a reasonable option. Many patients with dementia, with severe painful osteoarthritis of the hips and knees cannot tolerate larger doses of pain-killers such as narcotics which will make them more constipated and confused. When they get to the point where they can barely walk, the time has come either for permanent nursing home care and permanent immobility or an attempt to keep them mobile with joint replacement surgery. In a multi-disciplinary team setting this can be successfully done with appropriately selected patients.

## TESTING FOR DEMENTIA

There is no one specific test to diagnose Alzheimer's dementia. Many people are under the misperception that a brain CAT scan or brain MRI scan can diagnose dementia, but they cannot. However, on the brain scan when we see a lot of shrinkage (atrophy) of the frontal, parietal and medial temporal lobe (hippocampus) which is the memory centre, enlarged lateral ventricles which is the fluid-filled structures or intense white matter changes around the fluid spaces (periventricular white matter changes), these are all very abnormal findings which can correlate with a neurological decline such as worsening short-term memory and gait and balance disorders, although non-specific and not entirely diagnostic.

As a paradox, you can have Alzheimer's dementia with a fairly normal-looking brain CAT scan. However the more abnormal the brain CAT scan, the more likely there might be physical and cognitive signs that accompany it.

The best test in diagnosing dementia is a detailed collateral history from the patient's spouse, relative or close friend who knows them very well. The history of a progressive cognitive decline with worsening short-term memory and deteriorating function in day-to-day activities can help to diagnose the condition.

The patient should also have detailed cognitive testing which includes a formal memory test and cognitive testing of other domains of the brain such as thinking, which asks specific questions about-

- orientation in the day, date, month, year, season.
- where they are now.
- where they live.
- short-term memory and recall.
- problem-solving such as counting numbers backwards or spelling words backwards,
- writing a sentence with a noun and a verb that makes sense,
- reading comprehension test
- drawing a clock face accurately with numbers correctly spaced out and the correct time with hour and minute hands
- generating more than 11 words starting with the same letter within 60 seconds
- abstract reasoning and similarity testing
- concentration tests

The inability to draw the numbers correctly spaced on a clock face is a very sensitive screening test for cognitive decline. It is a warning sign that something is wrong and that further testing is needed. Also I find that those who call a picture of a rhinoceros a "Hippo" is very common in dementia but an unpublished observation. Again this is another warning sign that something maybe wrong.

Patients who do reasonably well on one memory test may generally fail on the more complex challenging tests, as they may test more specific tasks in several in domains of the brain and harder to pass in those with Alzheimer's dementia.

The typical clues that I see when testing someone's memory are:

- The patient's son or daughter are commonly very defensive and protective of their loved one. Therefore, they try to answer the questions for the patient. This is a very protective mechanism on the part of the relative and highlights the fact that they have not recognised the cognitive decline and assume that it is normal for the patient's age or are in denial.

- The patient looking towards the relative for the answer to the questions.

- Very peripheral in conversation and unable to answer questions directly, going off on a tangent.

- Unable to focus on the question or task at hand.

- Looking up to the ceiling and eyes flittering, as they are struggling to comprehend what is being said to them.

- Eyes closed, as they can't focus on the question with their eyes open due to easy distractibility.

- When asked what month it is, counting down the months of the year. This is common in dementia.

- Repeating the question to me instead of answering it as they just can't process the information themselves.

- When asked who the current Prime Minister is, they usually say "do you mean the one now". However, if they were asked who the Prime

Minister was in 1964 for example, they wouldn't have a clue.

- When asked who the Prime Minister is now, they commonly say "I know him, I can see him", but they can't name the PM. Or they say "I'm not interested in Politics" or "I don't worry about him.

- Unable to recount any recent news stories despite watching the TV news every night.

- Very slowed responses from impaired information processing.
- Inability to draw numbers correctly and accurately spaced out on a clock face.

- Limited verbal fluency and struggling to get words out.

- Simply not knowing why they are seeing the Doctor.

- Just being mentally slow and very vague.

Common patient response to memory testing include-
- Do you think I'm "mental"?
- This is silly!
- Do you think I am stupid?
- I'm not doing this!
- I didn't come to see you for this!
- I wasn't prepared for this!

Commonly sons or daughters will really compensate heavily for their elderly parents' deteriorating cognitive function.  They will say things like-
- "you have come on too strong" when I have asked the person where they live or

- "she wasn't prepared for that" when I asked the person what year it was or
- "she has had a busy day and is tired" when I have asked for their formal home address.
- Mum is always worse and more confused in the afternoon.

The son and daughter will also make a patronising or condescending comment such as
- "I couldn't answer that question myself" which is who the Prime Minister is or what year it is, to try and placate and reassure their elderly relative and to emphasise in their mind that it is okay to be forgetful when you are old, which it is not.

You've got to be kidding me! These relatives are highly functioning younger people operating businesses, driving cars, using computers, tablets and performing complex tasks on mobile phones, but they are not being honest when they say they don't know what year it is and who the Prime Minister is.

Let's get a reality check here! The human brain consists of about 100 billion neurones (nerve cells). Each neurone forms about 1,000 connections to other neurones, adding up to more than a trillion nerve connections! The brain neurones are a bit like the billions of grains of sand at the beach. If each neurone could only store a single memory, then the brain would run out of memory storage space rapidly. Although the brain has a limited storage capacity of a few gigabytes which is still a lot, similar to the space in a portable USB memory stick, neurones join together to store multiple memories at a time, exponentially increasing the brain's memory storage capacity to around 2.5 petabytes (or a massive million gigabytes!). So if your brain is compared with a hard drive recording video or an

SD memory card, 2.5 petabytes would be enough to store 3 million hours of music or movies! You would have to leave the TV or Tablet running continuously for more than 300 years to use up all that stored memory! So with so much brain power and memory reserve, there must be an almighty hit on brain function when someone starts forgetting simple things even with early mild Alzheimer's dementia. Even "mild" Alzheimer's dementia means that there is quite significant underlying brain disease to cause just mild memory impairment. Families will commonly say that their elderly parents' memory is much worse in the afternoon when they are tired, so that they shouldn't be tested then. How wrong can you be! That is the whole point! A normal elderly person's memory does not fade in the afternoon, nor do they get confused in the afternoon!

Having a new diagnosis of Alzheimer's dementia is a major threat to the relationship between a son or daughter and a mother. It is very threatening and sometimes frightening to think of the future consequences, loss of independence for the elderly relative and the need to provide more support for them. However, many of my patients with dementia can be safely and successfully supported at home with adequate medical care.

## MAJOR CAUSES OF CARER STRESS WITH DEMENTIA

- Afternoon and evening agitation- "Sundowning"
- Verbal or physical aggression
- Paranoid delusions
- Distressing visual or auditory hallucinations
- Wandering around the house or outside
- Night-time restlessness, pacing, insomnia
- Urinary and faecal incontinence

- Agnosia- loss of recognition of familiar faces, family and objects
- Anorexia- food refusal, not eating
- Argumentative
- Physical dependency with showering, toileting, and dressing
- Recurrent falls
- Unsafe driving

## DON'T TALK IN FRONT OF MOTHER

Many children are petrified of their older parents and refuse to discuss their mother or father's medical problems with them for fear of anger, retribution and negative outcomes. This is much worse with dementia. The family commonly warn me not to discuss Mum or Dad's memory loss and problems in front of their parents. This makes the consultation more challenging. Some of the reasons for this great fear of their elderly parents include-

-lifelong controlling and aggressive personality disorder.

-unresolved relationship issues.

-unreconciled love.

-worsening paranoid tendencies blaming children for everything going wrong.

-"gaslighting" , a form of emotional abuse by manipulating their children and forcing them to question their own memories, beliefs and undermining them by denying facts and reality.

-"guilt trip" and emotional blackmail by tormenting children to control them with statements such as "you just want to put me in a Nursing Home", "after all I have done for you", "you never phone me or visit me" when they already receive regular visits and phone calls.

Elderly parents with dementia can then become very difficult because they refuse help and advice when they are clearly struggling at home, and take out their anger and frustration on the family. Unless the tide can be turned, they end up in a crisis, crossing the "Thin Red Line" and then into the public hospital Emergency Department.

## **"WILL I GET DEMENTIA LIKE MY MOTHER"?**

Many sons and daughters are worried whether they will get dementia if I diagnose their elderly parents with dementia. The answer is generally "no". Most of the patients that I see are in their 80s and we call these sporadic age-related cases of dementia. The biggest risk factor for getting Alzheimer's dementia is increasing age but remember, only 25% of those over 80 have Alzheimer's dementia. If there are several elderly relatives in the same family with dementia, then there may be a higher prevalence within that family, but if they are over 70 they still may be sporadic cases.

It is only when there are 1st degree relatives with early onset of aggressive forms of dementia such as those below 60 years of age such as father or mother, and brother or sister, or other 1st degree relatives will the risk within the family be increased. There are genetic tests to see if you are at an increased risk for dementia such as the Apolipoprotein E (APOE) allele (variant form of gene).
The E4 allele of the Apolipoprotein E (APOE) gene is the main genetic risk factor for Alzheimer's dementia. APOE E4 carriers have an increased risk for brain amyloid angiopathy (accumulation of abnormal protein in the brain) and more rapid age-related cognitive decline during ageing. This is not normal ageing.

People with 2 copies of the E4 allele are at the highest risk. One E4 allele (heterozygote) gives a 3x increased risk of Alzheimer's dementia versus 2 copies of E4 (homozygous) increased the risk up to 12x compared with non-carriers of this allele. Although the APOE gene may increase your risk, it is not an absolute, definite risk for dementia. Patients who are homozygous for this allele are much more likely but not 100% definite to develop dementia. In addition, almost 40% percent of patients with Alzheimer's Dementia do not carry APOE. Given that this test is not 100% reliable one has to ask the question why would you want the test when you can't prevent it from happening, and at present the disease is not curable.

The best preventative measures to reduce the risk of dementia include-
- do not smoke,
- reduce alcohol consumption,
- reduce the number of sedative medications,
- avoid anti-cholinergic type drugs,
- avoid multiple general anaesthetics,
- avoid head injuries particularly in a sports environment,
- regular brisk walking exercises of 45 minutes a day,
- healthy Mediterranean diet with olive oil and grilled vegetables,
- colourful diet with lots of antioxidants including fresh fruits and berries,
- avoiding too much saturated fats, fried food and processed foods.
- Regular brain exercises such as cross-words, puzzles, word games,
- Regular social interaction.

## LIVING ALONE WITH DEMENTIA.

This is not a good situation to be in! The human brain needs mental stimulation to preserve neuronal connections and memories, and make new ones. Human beings are social beings and not meant to live alone, particularly in old age! The brain is a bit like a muscle- if you don't use it you lose it- muscles shrink and become weak without use, and so can the human brain unless it has social stimulation. Language skills, social interaction, and memory all decline when older people with cognitive impairment live alone. They tend to eat less, walk less and their dementia progresses more rapidly. Over time they may struggle with basic daily tasks such as shopping, cooking, managing medications, paying bills and organising their day. Even when community services come in for 1 hour 7 days a week to help, they are still alone for 23 hours a day!

Whilst we try to support and keep older people at home with dementia when it is safe and reasonable to do so, when they cross the "Thin Red Line" then they need to go into Residential Aged Care. These triggers for placement include inability to manage nutrition, hydration, medications, personal care, worsening incontinence, unsafe behaviours such as wandering or worsening agitation and distress. Unfortunately there are some families who are obsessed with keeping their very demented parents at home even when they are no longer able to look after themselves any longer. Then they are at risk at home alone of dehydration, malnutrition, falls, wandering away and elder neglect. Families will often say this is what Mum always wanted, to stay at home even when their Mother has lost capacity to consent to her place of living and life affairs due to advanced dementia. Some families even lock them in the house so that they don't wander away. We wouldn't leave or lock a 3 year old child at home alone, so why do some families still do this with their very frail elderly parents with advanced dementia?

## OTHER TYPES OF DEMENTIA

Apart from Alzheimer's dementia there is:

**Post stroke dementia**. This occurs after major cortical strokes and scarring in major parts of the brain. These patients with post-stroke dementia experience a stepwise cognitive decline after a stroke. They usually have prominent impairment of executive functions (planning and getting daily activites done), sometimes with relative sparing of memory. They may have other signs of stroke such as aphasia (comprehension and language impairment), dyspraxia (impaired co-ordination and planning of movements and activities), and apathy. This type of dementia can also cause memory loss and appear similar to Alzheimer's dementia.

**Vascular dementia.** Vascular dementia is dementia caused by a stroke or evidence of vascular brain injury on brain CAT scan or MRI scan. Many patients with Alzheimer's dementia already have evidence of previous strokes or vascular disease on brain scans without symptoms of previous strokes. The prevalence of vascular dementia is declining and is less than 10% of all dementia. Most vascular dementia is in fact Alzheimer's dementia or "mixed" dementia. Vascular dementia usually causes mild cognitive impairment only.
The risk factors for vascular dementia include-

* Smoking

- Hypertension
- Diabetes

- Coronary artery disease
- Atrial fibrillation (irregular heart rhythm)

- Elevated cholesterol levels

There have been dramatic improvements in population vascular risk factor control over the few decades, with substantial decreases in stroke incidence, so vascular dementia prevalence is also falling. So many patients are now on blood pressure pills, cholesterol pills, and blood thinners to prevent stroke.

Vascular dementia patients may have labile mood (pathological laughing and crying) slowing of walking, unstable bladder with incontinence, depression, impaired swallowing.

The usual cognitive impairment of Alzheimer's dementia differs from vascular dementia with more prominent impairment in short term memory in Alzheimer's. Vascular dementia patients usually have better recall and verbal learning but worse organising and planning skills. Unusual forms of Alzheimer's dementia, such as the "frontal variant", can make it difficult to distinguish from vascular dementia.

There are some questions whether vascular dementia is simply early onset stage of Alzheimer's dementia. Vascular dementia tends to be diagnosed when there are lots of these "white matter changes" around the lateral ventricles (fluid areas of the brain) on CAT scans or hyper-intense white matter lesions on brain MRI scans, but these areas may not be small strokes but rather an accumulation of abnormal protein including amyloid, scarring, degeneration of brain cells (neurones) and degeneration of blood vessels (hardening of arteries- arteriosclerosis). These white matter changes are commonly associated with memory decline, slowing up with walking speed, worsening balance and falls. The more prominent these white matter changes are (when they join up like a "ring of fire" around the lateral ventricles) on the brain scan, then the more risk of memory and balance decline. One of the big risk factors for having Alzheimer's dementia is in fact having a stroke or multiple strokes. I think that vascular dementia is way over-diagnosed! Most of these patients have in fact Alzheimer's dementia. It is commonly very difficult to distinguish between Alzheimer's and vascular dementia. Does it matter? Yes it does, as Alzheimer's dementia can be treated with drugs to slow down the progression of cognitive decline. I have never seen anyone with so-called vascular dementia get improvement in their dementia by treating vascular risk factors such as high BP, high cholesterol and diabetes! Many patients are hoodwinked by Doctors telling them that they "only" have vascular dementia, giving them a false sense of security. Then the family say it's OK, Dad "only" has vascular dementia! Most in fact have Alzheimer's dementia.

**Fronto-temporal dementia.** This is the name given to dementia due to degeneration or damage to the frontal and temporal lobes of the brain. These parts of the brain control mood, personality, social behaviour, attention, judgement, reasoning, planning your day-to-day living and self-control. The signs and symptoms of fronto-temporal dementia include personality change, becoming more withdrawn and socially isolated or hyperactive, impulsive, and lack of inhibition with socially inappropriate behaviour including rudeness and loudness in social situations, loss of empathy and understanding with others, poor judgement, repetitive compulsive behaviours including compulsive eating, inability to concentrate or plan different day-to-day activities, frequent and abrupt mood changes including verbal and physical aggression and deteriorating language with speech difficulties including understanding the meaning of words, finding words and getting the words out. Memory is generally unaffected in the early stages. Fronto-temporal dementia is very hard to treat. It is generally poorly responsive to medications such as anti-psychotics and sedatives to try and calm down aggression and agitation. It doesn't respond to the Acetyl Cholinesterase drugs which can slow down the memory loss in Alzheimer's dementia.

**Alcohol dementia.** Alcohol-related dementia can occur in those who consume excessive amounts of alcohol. It classically presents with very short-term memory and confabulations which means telling false stories and making things up. It classically affects short-term memory, with preserved long term memory and other cognitive functions.

**Wernicke-Korsakoff's syndrome** is related to Thiamine Vitamin B1 deficiency. Wernicke encephalopathy is a common, serious acute neurologic disorder caused by Thiamine deficiency. Its classical features are delirium (encephalopathy), oculomotor dysfunction (impaired eye movements), and gait ataxia (wide-based unsteady balance). This is a medical emergency as delay in treatment will result in permanent brain damage.

**Korsakoff syndrome** is a late complication of Wernicke encephalopathy. The typical features here are severe anterograde amnesia (loss of the ability to create new memories after the initial insult that caused amnesia while long-term memories from before that event remain intact), and retrograde amnesia (loss of memory for events that occurred before the onset of a disease). This occurs with excess alcohol consumption and after an acute episode of Wernicke encephalopathy.

**Thiamine Vitamin B1 deficiency** is common in elderly patients who consume excessive amounts of alcohol, particularly because of associated poor nutritional intake of calories and protein. Thiamine is essential for neurones (brain cells) to function properly. Malnutrition in the elderly can also cause nutritional encephalopathy and confusion through Thiamine deficiency.

**Lewy Body dementia.** This is a form of dementia similar to Alzheimer's dementia, but with associated visual hallucinations and Parkinsonism (slowing of movement, stiffness, shuffling and upper limb tremors similar to that seen in Parkinson's disease). There can be a fluctuating mental state and alertness. They may be agitated, very confused and hallucinating for some of the time and more settled at other times. The fluctuations can occur over a period of hours. They can develop extreme confusion, difficulty walking and settling at night. However, these features can also be seen in Alzheimer's dementia. These patients with Lewy Body dementia may also benefit from Cholinesterase inhibitor drugs, just like in Alzheimer's dementia. It is important in these type of patients that potent Dopamine-blocking anti-psychotics drugs such as Haloperidol or Risperidone are avoided when treating psychoses such as delusions, hallucinations and agitation, as they can make their Parkinson's-like symptoms of stiffness, tremor, shuffling and balance worse.

## **NON-DRUG MANAGEMENT OF DEMENTIA**

- Holistic multi-disciplinary care focusing on all the patient's medical, psycho-social and physical needs.

- Managing their other medical conditions, focusing on adequate nutrition, hydration and assessing swallowing.
- Safe swallowing sitting upright and forward to reduce the risk of silent aspiration and food and fluid going down the wrong way.

- Urinary incontinence management.

- Management of constipation and faecal incontinence.

- Pain management and keeping drug doses to the minimum.

- Assessing and managing mood and behaviour disorders.

- Regular exercise programme.

- Assessing falls risk in the home environment with home-based physiotherapy, occupational therapist and falls risk strategies there.

- Monitoring standing blood pressure and treating as appropriate if it drops, if causing postural dizzy symptoms and falls.

- Cognitive stimulation including referral to Adult or Dementia Day Centres and providing in-house respite to give carers a well-deserved break.

- Support for Carers including education programmes through the Dementia Carer Support Group and Residential Respite to give the Carers a well-deserved break to prevent Carer stress and Carer collapse.

- Refer to appropriate community services to support the person at home including assistance with personal care, housework and shopping as needed.

## DAUGHTERS IN DENIAL

Many children find nursing home placement of their parents with dementia very distressing. Daughters are traditional carers so I see this denial of dementia more commonly in daughters but sons can also be in denial. Many of the nursing home staff that I visit commonly tell me that families are in denial about the severity of their parents' level of confusion, the severity of their dementia and their care needs. This denial commonly leads to anger and frustration from the families and difficulties for the nursing home staff. It also compromises medical care of the elderly. The reasons for this denial include:

- No one has made a formal diagnosis of dementia.
- No one has discussed the dementia, its severity and the prognosis with family.
- Family do not want to hear bad news.

- Daughters want to maintain their relationship with mother and feel threatened by the diagnosis of dementia.
- Fear of losing control of the mother-daughter relationship.
- Unresolved guilt, unreconciled love and relationship dysfunction, with dementia threatening that relationship further.
- Fear of the unknown and future.
- Fear of losing their mother.
- They want their mother to live forever.

Common signs of daughter in denial about mother's dementia:

- Visiting the nursing home every day, "not letting go" and not accepting the diagnosis and nursing home care.
- Hovering around mother for hours, interfering in daily nursing care.
- Making multiple unreasonable demands on nursing home staff when mother is already having good care.
- Trawling through medical notes.
- Insisting that nursing staff report any changes in mother's behaviours and general condition even when there are only minor changes and mother remains stable.
- Making multiple unjustified complaints about care.
- Believing mother's untrue complaints when they have advanced dementia such as not seeing a doctor or nurse for weeks when they have daily care and regular doctor visits.
- Demanding changes to medications and treatment when the daughter is unqualified to make those decisions.

- Falsely believing that mother's dementia is mild because they can have a "nice" conversation. Many daughters will say to me "there are times when Mum can talk so well, can be so bright and clear, and remember so much about the past" despite their advanced dementia. The conversation is generally repetitive with little substance.
- Saying things like: "well there is nothing wrong with my mother!- she just has a lazy mind!" despite the fact that the dementia is so advanced.
- Insisting on full cardio-pulmonary resuscitation when mother has advanced dementia and multiple co-morbidities just because daughter wants mother to live forever irrespective of mother's quality of life and mother's wishes.
- Demanding copies of Doctors letters when they already know what is wrong with Mum just to show who is in control and not accepting the diagnosis.
- Complaining about a Geriatrician home visit referred by the GP to help improve the medical condition of Mum, which would be the best medical treatment mother could get, instead saying "Why wasn't I told about this!" because of fear of losing control of mother.
- Complaining that "I don't know what's going on" when Mum is in hospital despite being told exactly what the medical problems are. This is just to let everyone know the daughter is in charge (but fear of losing control of Mother).
- Daughter wanting the Doctor to report to her daily even though she is well aware of what is wrong with her mother.

- "There was nothing wrong with my mother until she came to hospital!" So we could just ask the question then why on earth is she in hospital in the first place! This is a show of anger and frustration at losing control of Mum in the hospital environment and not coping with her physical and mental decline.
- Angry about the diagnosis of dementia, saying that mother had a "hard day" and was "overwhelmed" when memory was tested, and you shouldn't be testing my older mother in the evening! Mother -Daughter relationship threatened by diagnosis of dementia.
- "You can't tell my mother anything when she is alone. She is old you know! I need to be there, but there is nothing wrong with her memory!"
- "My mother manages so well at home alone. She does everything for herself and remembers way back into the past." Yet her mother is confused, can't remember what happened yesterday and can't feed herself at home. Daughter phoning mother daily at home and checking on her anyway, and insisting on Doctors telling her what's going on, even though someone with normal mental function should be able to tell her daughter what's going on herself!
- Demanding to know every test result, every blood test result which the daughter can't interpret anyway, even though the Doctor would give an overall picture and let her know if there was anything major wrong.
- Demanding to know why a brain CAT scan was ordered without asking daughter when mother can still consent to this.
- Complaining that mother had a cognitive test to test her memory- "why would you ask a 90

year old lady such questions as where she lives just to upset her!"
- Daughter looking up the internet about medications prescribed by a Specialist and then deciding without any medical qualifications that Mother should not be taking that pill!
- Writing everything down on a clip board to intimidate the Doctors and Nurses to show who is in charge, for fear of not being in control and not accepting the diagnosis or treatment.

This denial usually results in carer and staff stress and limits what the nursing staff can do for the resident due to the unrealistic demands of family and the expectation now that family is always right, and the fear of formal complaints. Doctors and nurses commonly have to "manage" the daughter as well as the patient to placate the daughter to prevent nonsense, vexatious complaints to the medical board. Too many families are driving medical care for their elderly parents in hospitals and nursing homes without medical qualifications even when the parent is capable of making a decision about their own medical care.

Another common cause of family anger is when their elderly mother or father becomes immobile after suffering a prolonged delirium (confusional episode) after surgery or an acute medical illness. These elderly patients commonly had pre-existing dementia and walking/balance disorders not recognised by family nor previously diagnosed by the family Doctor. Then the family say that "Mum was quite sharp and nothing wrong with her memory till she got to hospital!" Then when the patient cannot stand and walk any more due to worsening confusion, dementia and underlying severe walking/balance disorder the family blame the Doctor and the hospital, and insist on "Rehab" as a magical cure when the patient is so impaired, de-conditioned and dyspraxic (confused with poor coordination and planning of movements) that they are beyond restorative care and remain immobile. They cannot participate in Rehab and in fact need Nursing Home Placement as a result of severe underlying neurodegenerative brain disease.

Of concern are families who refuse their elderly parents proper pain relief for severe pain when prescribed by the Doctor with unrealistic fear of morphine related side effects, even though the dose is low and the patient is carefully monitored. This borders on elder abuse through elder neglect of appropriate medical treatment. Why on earth would you refuse pain relief for anyone suffering severe pain?

Some families fill out the Advanced Care Plans for their elderly frail parents in nursing homes highlighting what medical treatment Doctors and Nurses should offer in an emergency situation when the person collapses from severe acute illness. However this should not be the daughter's wishes but the patient's wishes or at least what mother would have wanted if she was still able to voice that, to the best of the family's understanding of this. Many families insist on full CPR (cardio-pulmonary resuscitation) if mother has a cardiac arrest even with advanced dementia in a nursing home! This is the family's wish, not the patient's wish! To be brutally honest, this means crushing the chest, maybe breaking the sternum and ribs during CPR! It also means intubating and ventilating them (putting a tube down their throat, then onto a machine to help them breath and keep them alive while they are unconscious with very little hope of survival). Most frail elderly nursing home residents with advanced dementia and multiple co-morbidities would never survive a cardiac arrest, but it also raises the ethical question of why would you try to prolong the suffering of someone with advanced dementia anyway? Doctors in Australia are not obliged under law to provide unrealistic and futile treatment to patients when the burden of suffering is so great, the complications so severe, that the benefits are outweighed by the complications, suffering and poor outcome.

Families commonly like to take their mother out of the nursing home for an outing but when they return and drop them off, their mother frequently suffers disorientation, worsening confusion, agitation and general distress from the sudden changes in environment which they just can't cope with. The family feel good about the outing, their guilt is relieved and they feel that they have done a good deed for mother. However they are unaware of the distress and harm they are causing their mother with advanced dementia by these outings.

Denial is also a common reason why families insist on discharge from hospital against medical advice when mother has advanced dementia and doctors advise nursing home placement. Then their mother fails to manage at home and gets into a crisis, crossing the "Thin Red Line" and ends up in the public hospital Emergency Department.

The best way to help families cope with dementia is an accurate diagnosis and prognosis, and referral to the Dementia Carer Support group for counselling and support, and to learn about dementia and the behavioural and psychological disorders that complicate it. We should also be supporting older people with dementia at home with comprehensive community care packages when it is safe, reasonable and appropriate to do so.

# ACUTE CONFUSION/DELIRIUM

- Delirium is a sudden onset of confusion.

- It is a complex clinical syndrome characterised by acute onset.

- It always occurs abruptly over a period of hours or days.

- There is a fluctuating course. Symptoms tend to come and go with an increase and decrease in severity over a 24 hour period. There are characteristic lucid periods where the patient appears normal and then deteriorates, usually much worse at night with lack of sleep and then sleeps during the day.

- Usually is more severe in the evening when they become restless, wandering, agitated and wont sleep.

- Inattention.

- Difficulty focusing.

- Easily distracted.

- Difficulty keeping a track of what is being said.

- Disorganised thinking with unpredictable switching of subjects and unclear flow of ideas.

- Incoherent speech.

- Altered level of consciousness, sometimes alert and sometimes hyper-alert, then lethargic and drowsy but easily roused.

- It is a potentially life-threatening syndrome, as the underlying causes can be multi-factorial and it is usually associated with a severe underlying illness which is potentially treatable though.

- It is very common in the acute hospital situation with more than 50% of patients over 65 having some form of delirium which is commonly under-recognised, underdiagnosed and undertreated.

- It is common in both medical patients and in the post-operative surgical patient.

- It is largely ignored in the hospital and in the community. Unless it is looked for and screened, it is commonly missed.

- It is diagnosed solely on clinical grounds. There is no specific test.

- Delayed or missed diagnosis can result in early death of the patient.

- In fact delirium has a very high mortality and up to 50% of patients with delirium may die within 2-4 weeks as a result of the underlying serious causes.

- High rate of complications, in-hospital falls.

- Results in a loss of independence of the patient and a preventable massive increase in unnecessary health care costs to treat the complications of delirium.

- A reliable relative or friend is often needed to ascertain the time and cause of onset, as they can recognise the sudden change in cognition and personality of their loved one. Carers and family members usually have important information that can assist the Doctor and medical team with a diagnosis of delirium, particularly about the person's previous level of mental and physical functioning.

- While there can be significant cognitive impairments, they can still retain some brain function and recognise family during periods of lucid intervals. However, the confusion is typically global, with multiple deficits in brain function affected including orientation in time and place, memory deficits and difficulty getting words out.

- There are also marked perceptual disturbances, seeing insects or shapes on the wall, moving walls and other figures which can distress them. Visual hallucinations tend to occur in about 30%.

- There are also repetitive behaviours, picking at the bed sheets, very impaired sleep/wake cycle with daytime drowsiness and night time insomnia.

- Emotional disturbances with mood swings including fear, paranoia, anxiety, depression, irritability, apathy and anger which can be directed towards their family.

- There are other personality changes including new verbal and physical aggression, paranoid delusions which are commonly associated with resistive and aggressive behaviours towards family and nursing staff, agitation in a previously calm person, behaviours totally out of character or exaggerated pre-morbid personalities, so either a previously aggressive person will become more aggressive or placid and vice versa.

- There is also new wandering and intrusive behaviour and general disorientation.

- The delirium affects the whole of the brain function, so it can affect walking and balance. There can be dyspraxia or uncoordinated foot placement, slowing of movements, with a dramatic decline in walking and balance and high falls risk. The patient can become immobile with delirium.

- Autonomic dysfunction which means impairment of swallowing and co-ordination, with a silent aspiration risk of having pneumonia with food and fluid going down the wrong way, high blood pressure or low blood pressure, acute urinary retention, inability to pass urine which is a life-threatening complication requiring an in-dwelling catheter to decompress the bladder, constipation and even bowel obstruction.

- One of the most common signs of delirium is sudden onset of drowsiness. 95% of drowsy patients after surgery have delirium. Patients with post-operative delirium, with falls, slowing up and drowsy have the worst outcome. These are usually the sickest patients with more complications.

- There are 2 types of delirium: The hyperactive one about 30% who are overtly alert, increased agitation, restless, aggressive, paranoid, hallucinations and personality changes. About 25% are hypoactive, quiet, withdrawn, drowsy, lethargic and decreased level of movement, commonly misdiagnosed as depression with a very high morbidity and mortality. Mixed in 45%, fluctuating between the two.

Unfortunately delirium is missed in up to 2/3rds of cases, according to some studies. It is commonly misdiagnosed as dementia, resulting in inappropriate early discharge to a nursing home or a fatal outcome.

Delirium is a medical emergency! If delirium is diagnosed early, and the underlying causes found and managed in a multi-disciplinary care setting, then then full recovery is possible.

## WARNING SIGNS OF DELIRIUM

- Sudden onset of confusion.
- Worsening confusion in someone with known dementia.
- Not coping at home.
- Behavioural or personality change.
- Found on the floor.
- Unexpected new falls.
- Sudden deterioration in balance.
- Generally off and not quite right.
- New urinary or faecal incontinence.

In these situations delirium should always be suspected and the patient see the Doctor or present to the hospital Emergency Department as soon as possible.

# COMPLICATIONS OF DELIRIUM

- Falls.
- Dehydration.
- Aspiration pneumonia from food or fluid going down the wrong way.
- Malnutrition from poor dietary intake.
- Pressure sores from prolonged immobility.
- Infections
- Urinary retention
- Delirium itself is an increased risk factor for worsening underlying dementia.
- Delirium is a strong risk factor for new onset dementia in the older patients.
- There is a much higher risk of having a fall and hip fracture with delirium in hospital,
- Higher risk of ending up in a nursing home with delirium.
- Delirium can last between 1 week to 4 weeks. The longer it lasts the worse the outcome.
- Delirium is a common reason for hospital Emergency Department presentation of older people.
- Avoidable increased length of hospital stay.
- Increase health care costs.

# WHAT ARE THE RISK FACTORS FOR  DELIRIUM?

- Being over the age of 85.
- Commonly occurs after surgery in the elderly.
- Pre-existing memory loss, cognitive impairment and known Dementia.
- Functional impairment in day-to-day living including poor mobility and a history with falls.
- Other underlying neuro-degenerative walking and balance disorders.

- Background of stroke or Parkinson's disease.
- Pre-existing depression and other psychiatric illness.
- Infection is one of the commonest causes of delirium, either chest or urine infections.
- Adverse drug reactions, including to narcotic analgesics, pain-killers, Parkinson's medication, sedatives and anti-psychotic medications.
- Taking multiple medications.
- Low serum Sodium which can be caused by drugs such as SSRI anti-depressants, Thiazide diuretics including Indapamide and the HCT (plus components) of anti-hypertensives such as ACE and ARBs.
- Poor vision and hearing.
- Multiple chronic medical illnesses.
- Dehydration.
- Constipation.
- Urinary retention in itself can cause delirium.
- Urinary catheters.
- Following falls and head injury.
- Poorly controlled pain.
- Worsening heart failure.
- Worsening renal failure.
- Worsening liver failure.
- Heavy alcohol consumption or withdrawal from alcohol, sleeping pills or other medications, or a combination.
- Hypoglycaemia- low blood glucose.
- Worsening chronic lung disease-hypoxia-low oxygen levels.

## HOW IS IT TREATED?

- Comprehensive medical and physical assessments looking for reversible underlying causes for the delirium.

- Treatment of underlying medical conditions and infections.

- Review of medications.

- Particular attention to nutrition, hydration and early mobility.

- Expert management of bowel and bladder function.

- Supportive care in a multi-disciplinary care setting.

- Cautious use of low dose sedative and anti-psychotic medications for aggression, agitation and distressing psychosis (paranoid delusions, hallucinations).

- Unsafe wandering behaviour - may need to be managed in a safe, secure part of the hospital.

- Recovery can take days or weeks.

## HOW CAN FAMILY AND FRIENDS HELP?

- Speak to the Doctors and nurses first.

- Familiar objects around the bedside usually help and can reduce the duration and intensity of in-hospital delirium.  These include:
- A clock.

- A calendar.

- Family photos.

- Favourite magazines.

- Favourite music. Music therapy is very soothing and settling for agitated confused elderly patients.

- Favourite coat hanging up.

- Avoid large groups of visitors. Preferably visit in the morning rather than the afternoon when the agitation and confusion are generally worse.

- Avoid noise, too many people talking at once, overloading the delirium patient with too much information.

- Recovery may take days, sometimes weeks or months, but may occur more quickly with support of familiar friends, Carers and family.

- Family must remain calm with the patient suffering delirium, as arguments, excessive corrections and demands will worsen the patient's agitation and delirium. A calm reassuring approach is best.

Note that the brain CAT scan is usually normal in delirium, as the acute confusion is usually caused by something below or outside the brain, but impinging on the brain such as drugs and infection.

Consent is always an issue when the patient is acutely confused, but the Doctor out of necessity needing to treat a medical emergency dictates that delirium should be treated in an acute hospital situation which is necessary and reasonable to improve the health and well-being of the patient.

Of course we also like to discuss medical management plans with the family and carers and Enduring Guardian when available.

## NON-DRUG MANAGEMENT OF DELIRIUM

- Identifying and treating underlying medical causes.
- Stopping precipitating drugs and managing drug side effects.
- Ensuring good hydration and nutrition.
- Safe swallowing sitting upright and forward to reduce the risk of silent aspiration.
- Good mouth care with Sodium Bicarb mouthwashes, Lanolin to lips and Nystatin drops for oral thrush when necessary.
- Speech pathology assessment of safe swallowing.
- Correcting sensory deficits with appropriate hearing aids, glasses and adequate lighting.
- Re-orientation using a large clock on the wall, a calendar on the wall, personalised items including family photos, favourite magazines, books and favourite clothes hanging around them.
- A quiet environment, minimising staff changes in the hospital.
- Avoiding room and ward changes which can precipitate a worsening delirium through disorientation.
- Avoiding sleep disruption.
- Absolutely avoiding any daytime naps which will further worsen the sleep/wake cycle.
- A quiet, dark room with limited interruptions by staff to encourage sleep at night.
- the use of a high/low bed, as per guidelines, for patients with a high falls risk.

- Early mobility with physiotherapy to prevent the complications of prolonged bed rest and immobility.
- Active treatment of constipation to avoid urinary retention and bowel obstruction.
- Avoiding indwelling catheters in bladder unless absolutely necessary. The preference is to use in/out catheters in agitated patients.
- Involving family in the care setting to reassure and orientate the patient.
- Give the patient's family, relatives and friends a brochure explaining delirium and refer them to the local Dementia Carer Support Group to learn more about confusion.

## COMMUNICATION WITH PATIENTS WITH DELIRIUM

- Reassure the patient and family.
- Speak slowly.
- Get to the same level as the patient.
- Limit instructions, don't confront or argue and demonstrate what you want.

## "TOP 10" APPROACH

This means identifying with family the patient's favourite "top 10" items or routines that the patient likes to maintain. This includes what type of music they like, whether they like tea or coffee and what type of newspaper or magazine to help re-orientate them. This is also useful for patients with Alzheimer's dementia who are in care settings or in the unfamiliar acute hospital environment.

Patient's family and Carers are increasingly being recognised as important members of the "health care team".

## PREVENTING DELIRIUM

Targeting the risk factors, as above, and managing complications can prevent delirium or reduce the intensity and duration in hospital.

Unfortunately delirium is still allowed to be ignored both in the acute hospital setting and in the community. Doctors tend not to ignore an acute kidney injury and rising serum Creatinine (blood test) which reflects worsening kidney function, yet delirium is commonly not screened, identified or managed appropriately.

Delirium is everyone's business and ownership of the problem and attitudes to older people need to change rather than delegate this to just the "old aged specialists" or Geriatricians. All Doctors who look after the elderly patient should think delirium including surgeons and be constantly screening and looking for this very common problem in the elderly.

If delirium is screened for early, identified, diagnosed and managed early, the potential outcome can still be very good for the frail older patient.

# FALLS, WALKING AND BALANCE DISORDERS

- Whilst falls are very common in old age, not every older person falls regularly. Up to 40% of the elderly greater than 70 years report a fall in one given year. 50% of fallers experience multiple falls.

- The incidence of falls in the elderly rises steadily highest amongst those 80 years and over. Nursing home elderly residents have the highest falls risk - about 50% fall per year.

- Falls constitute 2/3rds of accidental deaths in the elderly and 75% of deaths caused by falls are those in patients over 65 years of age. The risk of falls related mortality dramatically increases with advancing age. Men have a higher death rate than women post fall, as they fall more violently. Nursing home residents over 85 years of age account in 1 in 5 fatal falls.

- Up to 30% of older people who fracture their hip after a fall die within a year of the fracture. Less than 25% of those elderly who fracture after a fall are on appropriate osteoporotic treatment which can reduce the risk of hip fracture in up to 50% of patients.

- 50% of older people sustaining a fractured hip never regain pre-fall level of mobility and function.

- Up to 25% of those with a hip fracture will end up in a nursing home within 12 months.

- Recurrent falls are a common reason for elderly people going into permanent nursing home care.

- recurrent post fall anxiety syndrome can result in self-imposed activity restriction and isolation at home for the older person.

## CAUSES FOR FALLS IN THE ELDERLY

Older people who fall are generally different from those elderly non-fallers in that they have impaired balance, they are generally frailer, they sway more when standing, they take more steps to turn around, they have impaired sensation in the lower limbs and they have weak quadriceps or thigh muscles and difficulty getting out of a chair.

Older people with recurrent falls are commonly on more medications including sedative medications.

Risk factors for falls include multiple medications such as sleeping pills, narcotic analgesia, anti-psychotic medications and cardiac medications causing a drop in blood pressure when they stand, causing dizziness. People using walking sticks or walking frames have a much higher risk of falls than those who walk independently without aids. Older people who fall usually have more than one risk factor. Most recurrent fallers have an underlying walking and balance disorder as well.

Public Hospital Emergency Departments tend not to sort out and diagnose the underlying causes of falls in elderly patients. They simply address whether there has been a major injury and if not, then send them home again to fall! No elderly patient who has had a major fall should be sent home from the Emergency Department until the causes of the fall are diagnosed and treated. One fall usually means they are at risk of further falls until sorted out! There are usually multiple causes for falls in the elderly which require comprehensive medical assessment, admission into hospital and multidisciplinary rehabilitation to prevent further falls.

## **"WIBBLE WOBBLE" OUT OF A CHAIR**

Muscle strength in the lower limbs is commonly impaired in recurrent elderly fallers. You can see them struggling to get out of a chair without using their upper limbs. Quadriceps weakness of the thighs is highly correlated with falls, as the thigh muscle is a very important stabiliser of standing balance and mobility.

When an elderly person can no longer get out of a chair without several attempts or needs to use their upper limbs to push them up, this indicates a very serious problem and a high falls risk. I commonly see these unwell elderly "wibble wobble" their bottom side to side sliding forward in the chair as much as possible, to the very edge of the chair, then rocking backwards and forwards several times, then leaning very heavily forward, to try and get out of the chair, almost falling flat on their face when they stand. It is usually associated with malnutrition, muscle weakness, wasting of the thigh muscles, an underlying balance disorder and very high falls risk. It is very important that this is properly medically assessed and diagnosed, as there is potential treatment to reverse the ongoing thigh muscle weakness and falls risk. Not being able to get out a chair quickly is a warning sign of serious problems.

## ELECTRIC TILT CHAIRS

I don't like these electric chairs where you press a button and they tilt forward to help push the person out of the chair. These commonly increase the risk for disuse muscle weakness and wasting because the person simply doesn't use their muscles when they are getting out of a chair. If you don't use it you lose it. The older person should always be encouraged to get out of a chair using their thigh muscles (quadriceps), as well as their upper limbs. Once they lose their quadricep thigh muscles and struggle to get out of a chair, then they are on the slippery slope downhill towards a fall at home, a long lie on the floor and complete immobility. It is a bit like the sinking of the Titanic. Unless the hole is fixed the ship will sink. Therefore, unless the muscle weakness is fixed they will fall.

## NORMAL OLDER WALKING PATTERN

Older adults maintain normal walking and balance patterns late into their 9th decade. Older people walk briskly and steadily with normal posture and balance without any help or walking aid! Ageing does not cause impairment of walking and balance. We must distinguish normal ageing from disease!

Many people believe that your walking slows up as you get older. No! No! No! No! No! You do not slow down as you get older. A well 90 year old can walk fast and as far as a younger person!

The typical but abnormal neuro-degenerative walking and balance disorder that I commonly see in the elderly and those who recurrently fall include a wide base of stance, smaller steps, diminished arm swing, flexed posture, flexion of the hips and knees, difficulty getting out of a chair, multiple steps with turning and generally unsteady without a walking aid.

These elderly people have great difficulty standing straight with their feet together, with a massive fear of falling and tending to go backwards with loss of balance. They can't do the heel/toe walk. Some of these patients with a flexed posture and slowed up will develop Parkinson's, but not all. The slowing of their walking and balance is a very reliable predictor of falls, increased risk for dementia and institutional care without a proper diagnosis, attention and treatment.

The typical history that I get from relatives is that I am usually told Mum or Dad have been slowing up with their walking for years, with a decreased stride length. This is abnormal and needs to be diagnosed and managed- the sooner the better!

## TIMED GET UP AND GO TEST

The timed get up and go test is a good predictor of falls risk in independently living older adults. The time taken to get up from a chair, walk 3 metres, get back and sit down again should be less than 14 seconds. More than this is associated with high falls risk. The slower they are the higher the risk of falls and confusion.

Elderly fallers are generally slower in their walking speed and have a shorter step length.
Limited slow and unsteady mobility significantly affects the independence of older people and their ability to manage the basic self-care (showering, dressing, toileting), and instrumental activities of daily living (shopping, cooking, housework, transport) necessary for independent living at home.

Poor mobility in older people predicts more general disability and susceptibility to other major Geriatric Syndromes. Those elderly who fall tend to have more car crashes.

## THE FORK TEST

Older frail people with neurodegenerative brain disorders are very slow in movements and reflexes. They lose their immediate safety reflexes to correct their balance if they are about to fall, so they can't save themselves from a fall. This is why they cannot drive a car safely. They are just too slow in thinking and movement. These people have a very high falls risk- low speed=high falls risk.

So when I see these frail older people in hospital and ask them to stand and walk when they are having lunch, they are unable to process the information quickly, they are unable to put their fork down, they just dither not knowing what to do, they need assistance to stand, they still hold their fork, and when starting to walk they still are incapable of putting their fork down on the plate even for a moment. They can't plan their movements. They have a very high falls risk. This is compared to a fit well person who would immediately plonk the fork onto the plate, stand up quickly and walk quickly.

## RISK FACTORS FOR FALLS IN THE ELDERLY INCLUDE:

- Severe arthritis of the hips and knees.
- Acute illness such as infections.
- Cognitive impairment and dementia.
- Parkinson's Disease.
- Previous strokes.
- Low standing Blood Pressure.

- Poor vision and hearing.
- Taking more than 3 medications.
- Narcotic analgesia.
- Anti-psychotic medications
- Long term steroids which cause proximal muscle weakness.
- Sleeping pills
- Cardiac medications causing a drop in blood pressure and dizziness when they stand
- other causes for low standing BP
- A previous history of falls indicates a high risk for further falls.
- Lower limb muscle weakness.
- Peripheral neuropathy or numb feet.
- Slowing up with a gait and balance disorder.
- Use of a walking aid.
- Sitting around all day.
- Difficulty getting out of a chair.
- Malnutrition with muscle weakness and wasting.
- Environmental factors such as poor lighting, loose carpets, mats and lack of bathroom safety equipment.

The risk of falls in the elderly increases dramatically as the number of risk factors increase. People with Alzheimer's dementia have a much higher falls risk due to confusion, poor co-ordination and planning.

Poor hearing and deafness increases the risk of falls, confusion, and depression. When hearing aids no longer work, a personal headphone amplifier may help at least with conversation (wearing headphones around ears and a microphone around the neck).

Many older women tend to cover perfectly good carpet with floor mats which have a high risk of trip hazard and falls. Their carpet will outlive them and not wear out long after they have gone! It is a common obsession with older ladies.

It is usually not recognised that malnutrition is also a potent cause of falls in the elderly due to muscle weakness and wasting of the lower limbs from poor calorie and protein intake.

Those elderly patients who are already using a walking stick or a walking frame have a much higher falls risk than otherwise normal elderly of the same age.

Those older people who lose height (they shrink) or have a flexed, forward curved thoracic back spine (kyphosis) already have advanced osteoporosis and have a very high risk of serious fractures with any fall. This osteoporosis must be treated to prevent it getting even worse and prevent fractures.

The biggest risks for falls in the elderly are acute hospital admissions and long hospital stays. Prolonged bed rest is a major contributor to falls, deconditioning, muscle wasting, pressure sores and falling blood pressure causing dizziness when the older person tries to stand up (postural hypotension). Early mobility with the Physiotherapist using a multicomponent exercise programme including balance, muscle strengthening, and weight bearing exercises has been shown to reduce falls in the frail elderly patient.

## MY FATHER HAS BEEN SLOWING UP FOR YEARS!

I see many elderly patients who have been slowing up, more unsteady with smaller steps when walking for years. They have recurrent falls. They struggle to get out a chair. Their exercise tolerance has drastically reduced from unlimited distance to only a few metres. They come to me very late because their family and their Doctor don't recognise that this decline in mobility is caused by serious medical illnesses and not "old age". These elderly patients can be helped and with a proper medical diagnosis and multidisciplinary treatment of their walking and balance problems, and commonly have spectacular improvements.

## I DON'T NEED MY WALKING FRAME!

Some older people have walking aids such as a walking frame with wheels or a walking stick. However many are stubborn and reluctant to use them! Many older people put their walking frame so far away from where they are sitting, instead of having the walking frame next to them. So when they get up to walk they struggle, stagger and shuffle over to the walking frame and risk a fall and injury! I see many older people who come into my consulting rooms without their walking aid. They say "it is in the car close by so I didn't need it". Falls can occur even walking short distances. Family members commonly yank them out of the waiting room chair then hang on to them arm in arm whilst walking when the older parent lives alone anyway and does not usually get any such help! Walking arm in arm is not a safe practice and increases the falls risk for these elderly people. In fact if the older person cannot get out of a chair on their own, then this is a medical emergency and requires hospital admission, a proper medical diagnosis to sort out why they can't get out of a chair on their own and holistic medical care by a Geriatrician to prevent falls, a long lie on the floor and a fractured hip! Walking to the shops without their walking aid and then hanging onto the shopping trolley is not a safe practice. Those elderly who tend to furniture cruise by hanging onto and leaning on furniture to get around the house have a very high falls risk! These people should have a proper medical diagnosis as to why they are wobbly and can't walk safely rather than just give them a walking aid. Those elderly who walk without their stick or frame any distance risk a fall, major injury and fractures!

## FAINTING AND BLACKOUTS (SYNCOPE)

Elderly patients who faint are at serious risk of major injuries and generally have a very high mortality (death rate) within 12 months of the faint when undiagnosed. Unfortunately witnesses can be very excited and emotional when seeing an elderly person faint. It is important to be able to diagnose the distinction between a fall, a "collapse" and becoming dazed and true unconsciousness after the fall.

**Unconsciousness:** Sudden loss of consciousness or syncope means a few specific diagnostic possibilities which include:

- A sudden drop in standing blood pressure, causing lack of blood flow to the brain (postural hypotension) causing syncope.
- Cardiac arrhythmia- either the heart rate is too slow or heart block or a very rapid heart beat, not able to maintain standing blood pressure.
- Seizure (epilepsy) without the classic features of shaking of the limbs.

Syncope sends a Doctor down a specific path of diagnosis and tests to exclude these life-threatening situations. However, most of the patients that I see have never actually fainted, but have had what relatives say "have had a collapse" and were "rushed" to hospital - very emotional terms. I call this the "movie star syndrome" where any famous person who suddenly falls is rapidly assisted and sent off to hospital for testing, when in fact they never lost consciousness. VIP's never fall or trip, they collapse!

Other causes of collapse include:

- Severe aortic stenosis (almost blocked aortic valve), limiting blood flow out of the heart.
- Carotid sinus hypersensitivity where the carotid artery receptor causes either low blood pressure or heart block, with movement of the neck which is a rare but important syndrome to exclude in the frail elderly who fall and lose consciousness without reason.

Other causes for falls include:

- Heart failure.
- Dehydration.
- Nocturia which is a major cause - getting up to the toilet frequently at night. Most falls in the elderly occur when getting up to the toilet at night. Therefore, their nocturia or recurrent frequency of urine at night should be investigated and treated to reduce their falls risk.
- Advanced Parkinson's disease in the elderly is associated with high falls risk and should be adequately treated and managed.
- The elderly with severe arthritis of the hips and knees have an increased falls risk. This can be managed with adequate pain relief, physiotherapy, rehabilitation and joint replacement surgery if needed.

## WALKING/BALANCE IMPAIRMENT WITH ALZHEIMER'S DEMENTIA PATIENTS

Alzheimer's patients in the medium to advanced stage commonly have walking and balance difficulties. This can be due to other causes or due to the dementia itself. They commonly have a cautious walking pattern in moderate dementia.

Frontal dementia patients commonly have disturbance of balance and mobility. Slowing up is very common, particularly in the more rapid or advanced stages of dementia. Progressive unsteadiness and asynchrony of balance with prominent rigidity of upper and lower limbs can be common.

The risk of falling is doubled in older people with dementia. They have a poorer prognosis once they have had a fall and are less able to make a good functional recovery after a significant injury, with a 5 times more likely risk of ending up in a nursing home than a non-demented elderly person.

Older people are much more likely to suffer severe injuries and multiple fractures after a fall. In the presence of a painful weight bearing joint after a fall, there is a fracture until proven otherwise, even with a normal plain X-ray. This is because of osteoporosis, fractures do not always show up on a plain X-ray in the frail elderly. They must have a nuclear medicine bone scan which is much more sensitive in picking up a fracture. However, it still may take at least 7 days for the fracture to appear on the bone scan due to slow reaction of osteoblast cells (bone producing cells) to show up the fracture in the elderly.

The mortality at 12 months after a fractured neck of femur is 3 times that of a cognitively normal elderly person of similar age.

## FALLS PREVENTION

Home-based physiotherapy has been shown to be the best intervention for reducing falls risk in the elderly. Interventions that help include-

- Lower limb strengthening exercises.
- Balance exercises.
- Medication review.
- Improving vision and hearing.
- Wearing safe footwear.
- Sorting out the nocturia, going to the toilet frequently at night.
- Occupational therapy home visit with installing ramps, rails, shower hoses, equipment and bathroom modifications to reduce falls risk.
- Measuring lying and standing blood pressure.

## HIP PROTECTOR UNDERWEAR

Wearing hip protector underwear with rubber cups on the side, on top of one's underwear can dramatically reduce the risk of hip fracture with falls. However, in my experience most older ladies are reluctant to wear them and generally have no insight into the risks they have for falls and hip fracture which can be a fatal condition.

Older patients who can manage to dress and undress and manage their underclothes should consider wearing hip protector underwear if they have a high falls risk. This is only after they have had an accurate diagnosis and a comprehensive assessment into the causes for their falls and treatment of any reversible factors to minimise their falls risk. Hip protectors need to be worn day and night, 24 hours a day for high risk fallers as 3/4 of all falls happen at night, particularly when going to the toilet.

## TWIST AND TURN

Almost all older people that I see walking with walking frames change direction and turn in an unsafe way. Their shoulder goes back, they lean back and twist to turn, taking multiple smalls steps increasing their falls risk. Instead, they should be changing direction with their walking frame by always walking forward in a large semi-circle like turning a big V8 car around, and always walking forward to reduce their falls risk. Turning and changing direction is a complex movement for people with walking and balance disorders.

## WALKING STICK VS WALKING FRAME

Many older people with serious walking and balance disorders refuse to use a walking aid to reduce their falls risk. Many prefer a walking stick to a walking frame. However, when their walking and balance is very impaired, then a walking frame gives much more support and safety when walking, particularly if the older person also has severe hip, knee or back pains. The walking frame takes the weight off their painful joints, gives them a wider base of support, reduces the falls risk, and allows them to walk further. Walking frames may also help the breathless patient to increase their exercise tolerance and distance walked. Of course the cause of the breathlessness must be diagnosed and treated first. Many older people just forget to use their walking frame thus increasing their risk for falls and fractures. So they need a diagnosis as to why they can't walk safely or get out of a chair unaided before we just give them a walking aid.

Remember, you wouldn't give a 21 year old person a walking frame if they suddenly couldn't walk so we shouldn't do the same to an 88 year old without a proper medical diagnosis as to the cause of their impaired mobility, and offer appropriate medical treatment!

# "TISSUE" SYNDROME

Most of the elderly ladies I see hang onto their tissues and won't let them go! Tissues contribute to falls and confusion in older women. Tissues can cause hip fractures in the elderly!

They are a distraction and cause sensory deprivation, particularly in those with cognitive impairments, Parkinson's disease and dementia. This relates to impaired "dual task interference" of being able to do two things simultaneously when there is cognitive impairment. For example, if you ask a cognitively impaired older person to walk and count the months of the year backwards, they tend to freeze and do only one task at once. The same thing happens with holding a tissue. This can distract them and increase their falls risk.

Frail older people with cognitive impairment should not be holding onto tissues or hankies with walking and should concentrate on focusing on using their walking stick or walking frame appropriately.

There are 3 types of "Tissue Syndromes"-

- Type A- they give up their tissue fairly quickly when asked without too much fuss- this group has the lowest but still increased falls risk.

- Type B- they struggle to give up their tissue when asked, very slow, "dither", become agitated, and not sure where to put it down- this group has a moderate falls risk.

- Type C- they are unable to give up their tissue when asked, and refuse to let it go, become agitated, and distractible, - this group is more likely to unsafely bend over and pick up tissues and other objects from the floor with a very high falls risk and are usually the most frail and the most confused. They do worse than the other 2 groups and usually need nursing home placement.

# THE "WOOZY, GIDDY, HEADY, DIZZY" PATIENT

Older patients who complain of these non-specific symptoms commonly have either:

- A walking and balance disorder which gives them a perception of dizziness, when they have a fear of falling and uncertainty with balance.
- Postural hypotension which is a drop in their standing blood pressure due to drugs or autonomic neuropathy from dementia, causing dizziness when they stand.
- Arthritis, chronic pain and anxiety including arthritis of the cervical spine (neck vertebrae) which gives them a sense of unsteadiness or dizziness in a non-specific way.
- Middle ear disease causing vertigo and disequilibrium with changes in posture or just turning the head
- Cerebellar disease (back of the brain) which controls balance

Most woozy, giddy, heady and dizzy elderly ladies that I see have a multitude of symptoms causing this including adverse drug reactions, low blood pressure, a walking and balance disorder, chronic anxiety and depression and/or cognitive impairment.

# POSTURAL HYPOTENSION

Postural hypotension (orthostatic hypotension) is one of the commonest causes of falls in the elderly. This syndrome is a sudden drop in standing blood pressure when the patient transfers from sitting to standing, thus causing dizziness, reduced blood flow to the brain and falls. It can also result in sudden confusion, unconsciousness and major injuries such as hip and other fractures.

While it is a very common problem in the elderly, it is commonly ignored, under-recognised and undertreated. It can occur in up to 50% of hospital inpatients over 75 years of age. It can lead to severe dizziness, fainting and injuries.

It is often multi-factorial in origin due to many different reasons, the commonest being:

- Adverse drug reactions from heart medications.
- Blood pressure pills lowering the blood pressure too much.
- Autonomic neuropathy from degeneration of the brain stem which supports standing blood pressure.
- Dehydration.
- Severe anaemia.
- Severe heart failure and other medical conditions.

It can be identified by measuring the blood pressure in a lying position and then after the patient has been standing for 3-4 minutes.

The lying and standing blood pressure should be routinely measured in all elderly patients.

Unfortunately over the years I have had great difficulty getting the nurses and Doctors to routinely measure the lying and standing blood pressure unless it is written down on the observation charts.

As the normal human position is in the upright posture, we should always be measuring the standing blood pressure. Unfortunately it is deemed too difficult and too time consuming, so the simplest option is just to take the sitting blood pressure which is the wrong approach. I frequently see catastrophic drops in blood pressure when the patient stands up which can contribute to confusion. This can be treated. The culprit medications can be reduced and the patient can stop falling.

I was one of the first to publish on this - "Overlooking Orthostatic Hypotension in the Elderly" (Australian Journal of Ageing, V21:2002; p213) Ref 26. Even now, blood pressure in hospitals and in the community is still taken incorrectly much of the time by Doctors and nurses.

## HYPERTENSION IN THE ELDERLY

There is well established evidence-based medicine that actively treating hypertension (high blood pressure) in the elderly significantly reduces the risk of heart attack and stroke. Treatment of high blood pressure also reduces the risk of chronic kidney failure and may reduce the risk of dementia. The elderly have the most to gain from these active treatments as stroke and heart failure after heart attack can be very disabling for the older patient and may result in permanent dependency on outside help to remain at home or in fact may result in nursing home placement.

The target blood pressure readings for hypertension treatment are constantly being lowered by new research studies. However, these studies may not always include the type of frail elderly patients whom I see, and may under-report the drug side effects of blood pressure pills and not report postural hypotension.

Blood pressure pills are one of the commonest causes of adverse drug reactions and falls in the elderly.

The current recommended blood pressure target level for older patients and those elderly patients with heart failure, diabetes or kidney failure is around 130/80 or lower. This maybe too severe for the frail elderly. Serious adverse events from blood pressure pills including very low blood pressure (hypotension) syncope (fainting), bradycardia (very slow heart rate) or arrhythmia, hyperkalaemia (high serum potassium), and renal failure occurred significantly more frequently in the more intensive versus standard blood pressure treatment groups.

I generally take a less aggressive approach to blood pressure lowering in the frail elderly, as although they may still benefit from blood pressure treatment, the risks of adverse drug reactions, postural hypotension and falls is much higher. Blood pressure treatment should be individualised in the frail older patients with the goal of minimising drops in standing BP (postural hypotension) falls, and confusion.

The take home message is that blood pressure must always be taken lying then standing to exclude significant postural hypotension.

# SWOLLEN ANKLES

Swollen ankles are common in older patients, but are abnormal.  They are not a normal part of old age!

Your ankles should not swell as you get older, even when you are 100!

Swollen ankles tend to bother older ladies, but they are commonly asymptomatic (they get no pain from them).

The commonest causes of swollen ankles are:

- Dependent oedema from lack of walking and sitting around all day, just like on a long plane flight.  This is caused by impaired circulation including venous and lymphatic return of fluid. The treatment of this includes a regular exercise walking programme to pump the fluid out of the legs, leg elevation when not walking and support stockings which are not too tight, but help to compress the fluid upwards.

- Another major cause is unrecognised heart failure, causing leg swelling.  Ankle swelling may be the first sign of heart failure.  This should be properly investigated and treated including with a detailed clinical examination, chest x-ray, ECG and echocardiogram.

- Malnutrition is also a common but under-recognised cause of ankle swelling in the elderly. Those elderly who have inadequate intake of protein and calories can eventually get a low level of albumin (serum protein) in the blood which helps to keep fluid in the blood vessels.  With malnutrition the liver which normally produces protein can't keep up, so the combination of a lack of protein synthesis in the body, lack of protein (serum albumin) keeping fluid in the blood vessels allow it to leach out into the ankles.

- Another cause is protein loss in the urine from progressive kidney failure and protein loss from progressive liver failure. This causes fluid to leak out into the tissues.

- Underlying cancer with malnutrition.

- Unilateral (only one) leg swelling could be associated with a clot in the leg, although it is very hard to diagnose a DVT (venous thrombosis/clot) without a Doppler ultrasound examination.

- Pulmonary emboli (blood clots on the lungs) can be a silent cause of worsening lower limb and ankle swelling. Pulmonary emboli usually present with chest pain and breathlessness, but in older people they can just present with lethargy, lack of energy and swollen ankles. The risk factor of this is particularly in older ladies who sit around all day, don't drink much and don't walk much.

## HEART FAILURE

Heart failure prevalence increases with age. About 10% of people over 80 years have heart failure but that means the majority do not! Improved treatment of heart disease and high blood pressure mean that people are now surviving into much older age before they develop heart failure. Heart failure can be categorised into 1/3 who have heart failure with preserved ejection fraction (HFpEF) and 2/3 with heart failure with reduced ejection fraction (HFrEF).

HFpEF increases with age due to stiffening of the heart muscle and failure of heart muscle to relax (causing back pressure in the lungs with fluid retention). Heart failure commonly causes ankle swelling, loss of energy and lethargy, weight gain from fluid retention, breathlessness on effort, reduced exercise tolerance, dizziness, breathlessness lying flat in bed and breathlessness waking the person up at night (PND-paroxysmal nocturnal dyspnoea).

HFrEF occurs when the heart muscle is weakened by previous heart attacks, leaking heart valves, long standing untreated high blood pressure or cardiomyopathy (disease of heart muscle).

Heart failure is worsened by other acute illnesses such as chest infections, rapid heart rates, anaemia and iron deficiency. Poor controlled AF (rapid atrial fibrillation irregular heart rhythm) can also tip an older person into worsening heart failure. A weak heart does not tolerate rapid heart rates.

Heart failure can cause confusion, low blood pressure and falls in the elderly. Low blood pressure commonly limits how much heart failure treatment an older person can tolerate.

Treatment of heart failure commonly involves diuretic tablets such as Frusemide, other cardiac pills to lower the blood pressure and heart rate, drinking less fluid (fluid restriction) and low salt diet. Renal function needs to be carefully monitored as fluid restriction and diuretics can cause kidney failure. There must be a careful balance between treating symptoms of heart failure and worsening renal function. If blood pressure is lowered too far with treatment then this can increase the risk of falls, lethargy and confusion.

## LOW SALT DIET

Eating salty foods makes you more thirsty and causes the body to retain more fluid. Eating a low salt diet is not easy as most of our packaged, processed and takeaway foods are caked in salt! We eat far too much salt! A low salt diet is less than 50mg a day. Even a small 185 gram can of tuna can have as much as 888mg of salt! A 500 gram jar of tomato paste has 2300mg of salt! A 150 gram packet of chips has at least 714mg of salt. Biscuits, breakfast cereals, frozen meals, processed sauces, chips, snack foods can have a lot of salt in them! You could end up eating your entire monthly salt intake in just one meal with these highly salty foods! Basically if the food is processed and in a jar, plastic or cardboard package then it is usually caked in salt!  You really have to read the label. The only low salt food is that which you cook fresh yourself. Lemon juice is a good substitute for salt.

# THE BREATHLESS OLDER PATIENT

People do not get breathless as they get older!
Exercise tolerance in 90 year olds should be unlimited.

Unfortunately many families incorrectly assume that their relatives become breathless as they get older. Therefore there is a delay in diagnosis in seeking out treatment for potentially treatable and reversible conditions.

Any new onset of breathlessness or decline in exercise tolerance in an older person may indicate an acute or chronic illness which needs to be accurately diagnosed and managed. While Doctors may not be able to fix all causes of breathlessness, in most cases we can do something to reduce symptoms, depending on the diagnosis.

There are many causes of acute and chronic breathlessness. If the patient's onset of breathlessness is sudden and severe they should be seen in the hospital Emergency Department to diagnose and exclude life-threatening conditions. These include:

- Heart attack.
- Angina from coronary artery disease.
- Pulmonary embolus or clots on the lung.
- An acute chest infection.
- Heart failure.
- Lung collapse.
- Exacerbation of known emphysema or smoking-related chronic lung disease.

- Anaemia (a low haemoglobin which is the oxygen-carrying capacity of red blood cells).

Sudden breathlessness in a patient with dementia or Parkinson's could represent silent aspiration pneumonia from food or fluid going down the wrong way due to swallowing incoordination.

Chronic breathlessness could be related to heart failure or chronic underlying lung disease such as emphysema. Older people must stop smoking as there are still big health benefits in quitting smoking even over 80 years of age! You are never too old to stop smoking!

Severe calcific aortic stenosis (a blocked main aortic valve in the heart which pumps the blood and oxygen out of the heart) can cause breathlessness on effort in the elderly without chest pain.

Heart block with a very slow heart rhythm can cause dizziness and breathlessness.

A rapid irregular heart rhythm such as rapid atrial fibrillation or other fast cardiac arrhythmias can cause breathlessness on minimal effort, as the heart can't pump enough blood and oxygen out.

Acute or chronic breathlessness causing disabling impairment of exercise tolerance is always a concern and needs to be appropriately managed and treated. It has nothing to do with old age!

All of these conditions are potentially treatable in the elderly, but depend on the extent of the pre-existing underlying lung disease present.

It is important to note that we would not accept a 21 year old man having sudden breathlessness or worsening chronic reduction in exercise tolerance, yet many people feel that for a 90 year old it is okay to be breathless when there are potential treatment options available. Would we say to a 21 year old- "yes you are breathless but you are 21 years old you know!" Then why do we say- "well you are 90 you know- what do you expect?"

# CHRONIC PAIN

Chronic pain is very common in older patients. It is usually underdiagnosed and undertreated. It has enormous impacts on day-to-day function, mobility, falls risk and quality of life. Over 50% of elderly suffer from some form of chronic pain.

In terms of chronic arthritic pain of the hips, knees and lower back, narcotic (opioid or morphine) analgesia has revolutionised the management of chronic pain in the elderly. These days the use of low dose narcotic analgesic oral medications or pain patches has helped control severe chronic pain in the elderly. The patient should be adequately informed of the potential for adverse drug reactions with narcotics including nausea, drowsiness, constipation and confusion. These side effects may not appear for 7 to 10 days until the drug level has built up in the body. The dosage should always be started off in a very low dose. The patients most at risk of narcotic side effects include those with severe frailty, malnutrition, dementia, chronic heart failure, severe chronic lung disease and kidney failure. There is a risk for long term dependency, but commonly the benefits may outweigh the side effects in maintaining mobility and quality of life.

There is increasing difficulty for Doctors to be able to prescribe pain killers for older patients. There are increasing Government and bureaucratic controls on narcotic analgesia with limits on what can be prescribed and for how long, resulting in reluctance to prescribe. However appropriate pain control results in improved mobility, falls reduction and better quality of life. Chronic pain in the elderly is associated with an increased incidence of adverse outcomes, including impairment of daily general function, falls, depression, impaired sleep and decreased appetite. Older people have an increased risk of adverse drug reactions with pain killers which can also interact with other multiple pills that they are taking. Therefore the dose of pain killers should always start low and the patient should be regularly monitored for side effects.

Elderly patients may benefit from guided injections into arthritic painful shoulders, hips, knees and lumbar spine with sciatica for temporary pain relief.

Chronic nerve pain pills such as Gabapentin or Pregabalin can assist in the management of painful nerve pain in the lower limbs and back, and post herpetic neuralgia (shingles nerve pain) but for every 9 treated patients with these drugs, one will get severe side effects including drowsiness, worsening balance and falls. Again the dosage should be very low, but in combination with a comprehensive Geriatric Medical review, physiotherapy to improve balance and lower limb strength and review of all other medications there can be significant improvements in chronic pain. Patients with chronic low back pain and lower limb arthritic pain can be successfully managed and regain independent mobility.

There is a role for joint replacement surgery in painful arthritic hips and knees in the elderly patient when physiotherapy and oral medications are no longer effective. Older people have the most to gain in reducing falls risk and injury and preventing early nursing home entry when they were functionally independent prior to surgery. Older people can also benefit from spinal surgery when they have severe unmanageable back pain and sciatica that either doesn't respond to reasonable doses of pain killers or they just can't tolerate the side effects of pain medications.

There is no age limit for surgery provided the older patient is fit for anaesthetic and surgery, and will benefit from it to improve chronic symptoms, mobility and quality of life.

Many older patients do not have adequate treatment for their chronic pain. The cause of the chronic pain must of course be diagnosed accurately first, as the underlying cause may be treatable without the need for chronic pain medications.

I still see some frail elderly patients whose families are reluctant for them to have proper treatment for their pain! Can you believe that! Families do not want their mother or father to have pain relief! This is elder abuse and relates to uninformed views that pain killers are bad for older people, particularly morphine and other narcotic analgesics. The risks of drug addiction is irrelevant when taking low doses carefully prescribed and monitored by the Doctor. With informed consent about potential side effects most people want pain relief. Anyway, a Doctor has a duty of care to treat severe pain.

# URINARY INCONTINENCE

Urine or faecal incontinence is NOT a part of old age or normal ageing. Most older people are still able to control their urine and bowel function effectively.

Nevertheless, incontinence is a very common problem in the elderly. More than 33% of people over 80 years have some form of incontinence and overactive bladder. It is twice as common in elderly women. The figure is much higher is nursing home elderly. Remember then, that about 70% of the elderly do not have incontinence! However, people over 85 years of age are 5 times more likely to experience severe incontinence compared to people under 85 years. It can be very disabling and negatively impact on the quality of life of older people, their level of independence and social interaction.

As you get older the bladder volume at which it signals that you want to void is lower. You can't hold as much volume of urine and you may want to go a little more often than a younger person. However, unstable irritable bladders in males and females can be very distressing and disabling and contribute to falls risk particularly a night. An unstable bladder is a sudden urge to void small volumes of urine without warning which can contribute to urinary incontinence.

In females the common causes of an unstable bladder include a neurological condition such as Parkinson's disease, stroke and dementia. In males they have similar problems, but it also can be caused by the prostate which can enlarge, reducing urine flow and causing an irritable bladder.

In any older patient with an unstable bladder it is important to measure the bladder residual urine volume (how much is left after a good wee) to make sure the bladder is emptying and not in acute or chronic urinary retention. This can be done with an ultrasound examination.

If the bladder won't empty and develops chronic retention, the patient could develop back flow pressure which could cause swelling of the kidneys (hydronephrosis) and eventually chronic renal failure.

If the patient develops acute retention sometimes it is painless, but can contribute to confusion and falls and increase their risk for urine infections and delirium. In males with an enlarged prostate causing an unstable bladder, it is again important to rule out acute on chronic retention of urine with a renal tract ultrasound and prostate cancer with a digital rectal examination and serum PSA.

The options for treatment of prostatism and an unstable bladder in the elderly include medical therapy first before surgery.

Older patients with poorly emptying bladders which are irritable should avoid constipation and anticholinergic drugs which will further impair bladder contraction and may result in acute urinary retention which is a medical emergency requiring an indwelling catheter.

New urinary incontinence in an older patient may be the first sign of delirium. A urine infection in the elderly does not usually result in incontinence, but rather causes confusion and falls.

Urine infections in the elderly are commonly asymptomatic. In other words, they don't always get urinary frequency, going more often and burning, but rather they feel unwell or develop delirium.

## CHANGES IN BLADDER FUNCTION IN OLDER AGE-

Changes in the lower urinary tract with older age that increase the risk of incontinence include:

- Bladder muscle overactivity
- Increased volume of urine produced at night
- More bacteria in urine
- Weaker bladder contractions
- Reduced bladder sensation of fullness
- Reduction in bladder volume- holds less urine
- Less warning to pass urine
- More getting up at night- nocturia

Urine incontinence could be caused by bladder storage problems-

- going more often, particularly at night,
- frequency,
- urgency with little warning,

or voiding (passing urine) difficulties-

- hesitancy
- poor urine flow
- dribbling after finishing
- needing to strain
- dysuria (burning)

Whilst prostate enlargement increases with age, not all older males have symptoms or problems with urine flow.

## CAUSES OF URINARY INCONTINENCE:

- Multiple chronic medical conditions
- Cognitive decline
- Dementia
- Delirium
- Multiple medications
- Constipation
- Enlarged prostate
- Diuretic medication for heart failure
- Diabetes
- Parkinson's Disease
- Strokes
- Sleeping pills

An enlarged prostate can cause obstruction to urine flow and an irritable over active bladder. However up to 50% of elderly men may have a weak bladder muscle (hypo-contractile detrusor) causing poor bladder emptying and poor urine flow. This has treatment implications because bladder relaxant drugs used to treat a presumed overactive bladder may make this worse. Over active bladder is common in strokes, Parkinson's Disease and dementia. The brain loses control of the bladder, so when the bladder fills just a little, the person has the urge to pass urine but can't get to the toilet quick enough. Diabetes can cause nerve damage to the bladder resulting in a poorly emptying bladder. Heart failure patients on diuretic medication can have problems with incontinence from fluid overload and the effects of the heart medications.

## NEW ONSET URINARY INCONTINENCE-

Note that sudden onset of new urinary incontinence in an older person is always abnormal and a serious problem- it may reflect underlying new acute medical problems such as infection outside the urinary tract, delirium or a new adverse drug reaction. Acute urinary retention with overflow incontinence appearing suddenly as an unstable, irritable bladder, with a constant dribble must always be considered in an older person with acute new onset urinary incontinence. Without diagnosing acute urinary retention, the patient may develop back pressure into the kidneys (hydronephrosis-swollen kidneys), kidney failure and serious infections. This requires urgent medical attention and sorting out. It usually requires an indwelling urethral catheter to decompress (empty) the bladder. Then the cause of the acute retention needs to be diagnosed and treated. Urinary tract infections uncommonly cause incontinence in the elderly. Rather they can cause delirium and falls. Urine infections can make patients with Dementia more agitated.

Older people with incontinence are generally frailer, take multiple medications, have cognitive impairment, history of falls, walking and balance disorders.

## GETTING UP FREQUENTLY AT NIGHT-

Getting up frequently at night to pass urine (Nocturia) is one the commonest causes of falls in the elderly. Nocturia and incontinence should be actively investigated, diagnosed and treated in the elderly to improve quality of life and reduce falls risk. Control of underlying diabetes, heart failure and reducing fluid intake and caffeine in the evening may help. Bladder anti-spasm drugs may help but bladder emptying needs to be assessed first with an ultrasound scan to measure retained urine volume from incomplete bladder emptying. Retained urine volume in the bladder can increase with these type of drugs thus increasing the risk of urinary tract infections. There is also the risk of urinary retention in men with enlarged prostates.

Passing blood in the urine is always abnormal and should be investigated- one must suspect bladder cancer here until proven otherwise. Other causes include bladder stones, bladder polyps, kidney cancer and less likely infections.

Lower urinary tract symptoms in older men is usually due to an over active bladder or prostate enlargement. In older women it is usually due to weak muscles of the pelvic floor or overactive bladder.

## MANAGING URINARY INCONTINENCE-

There are several approaches to helping the elderly with urinary incontinence including-

- renal bladder ultrasound to assess kidney/prostate size and bladder emptying
- blood test of kidney function
- urine culture to exclude infection
- bladder diary to establish pattern
- restriction of fluid intake at night
- pelvic floor exercises
- bladder retraining/prompted voiding routines
- urodynamic studies to measure bladder pressure/volume/emptying and urine flow
- drug treatment
- assessing the safety of toilet access at home
- providing extra support services at home/Carers

Non-drug treatment is the first and preferred option. However, anticholinergic drugs are commonly used to treat over active bladder in the elderly, but they have a very high side effect profile including-

- confusion
- dry eyes and mouth
- constipation
- blurred vision
- worsening glaucoma
- acute urinary retention- this is an emergency requiring an indwelling catheter to drain/decompress the bladder.

Constipation in the elderly is a common but treatable cause of bladder dysfunction, urinary incontinence and urinary retention.

Some drugs used to treat prostate enlargement/outflow obstruction such as Tamsulosin and Prazosin can cause low blood pressure in the elderly and increase falls risk. Sedative drugs and sleeping pills such as benzodiazepines, anti-psychotics, and diuretics can worsen bladder control and incontinence.

Overall urinary incontinence can be managed and improved in a significant number of elderly patients, particularly if they receive multi-disciplinary care to improve their nutrition, mobility and reduce the number of medications that they are taking.

## CATHETERS AND SPC

Urinary tract catheters increase the risk for delirium, falls and urinary tract infections in the elderly. They should be avoided unless absolutely necessary or if the person is in acute urinary retention or immobile with flooding urinary incontinence causing sacral pressure ulcers. If a long term urinary catheter is required then an SPC (Supra Pubic Catheter) is a better option as it is better tolerated than a urethral catheter and less risk of urinary tract infections. An SPC is surgically inserted through the skin in the lower abdomen under local anaesthetic directly into the bladder. Catheters should be changed by a nurse every 6 weeks. To prevent recurrent urinary tract infections the person with a catheter should drink lots of fluid, and the urine should be acidified with Vitamin C tabs, Hexamine Hippurate tabs and Cranberry tabs.

# DIABETES

In my experience, diabetes is generally over-treated in the frail elderly. The purpose of treating diabetes in the elderly is to avoid very high blood sugars and a hyperosmolar, non-ketotic state which means severe dehydration and delirium. The build-up of acid from high sugars (ketoacidosis) is very uncommon in the elderly.

Appropriate treatment and control of blood glucose levels in younger patients to prevent long term vascular complications such as stroke, heart attack, microvascular kidney disease, kidney failure and peripheral vascular disease including leg ulcers and gangrene requires a fairly "tight" diabetic control over many years. However, in the elderly these issues are not as important as simply preventing hypoglycaemia or a low blood sugar less than 6.

Hypoglycaemia is commonly asymptomatic (the patient is not aware of the low blood sugar), but this can cause confusion (delirium) and falls, worsening of their dementia and worsening of their gait and balance.

Therefore, in frail older patients, particularly those with multiple co-morbidities or other disease processes and dementia, I tend to be very conservative with blood glucose control. While ideally the blood glucose should be between 6 and 12, sometimes I will allow the blood glucose to go up to 14 or even higher if necessary, simply to prevent hypoglycaemia which can be catastrophic for these types of frail patients. Hypoglycaemia destroys brain cells.

Diabetes in the elderly should be carefully managed and treatment should be individualised for the frail older patient to absolutely avoid hypoglycaemia less than 6.

## **DIET FOR OLDER PEOPLE WITH DIABETES:**

Older people and their families think that diabetic elderly literally have to starve and drastically reduce kilojoules just because they have diabetes. I still see many malnourished elderly diabetics! Malnutrition is equally important in diabetic elderly as it is in non-diabetic elderly.

It is important to have a low GI carbohydrate at each meal and have regular meals times. It is also important to make sure you are eating enough food, including kilojoules for energy and protein to prevent muscle breakdown. Elderly diabetics should not skip meals! They also need regular snacks between meals.

Diabetics who are malnourished need to eat more of the right food including extra protein, low GI foods rather than eating less.

## **CARBOHYDRATES:**

- Too many carbohydrates at each meal can increase the blood glucose levels. High GI foods such as chocolates, biscuits, cakes, chips, ice cream, fruit juices, soft drink (soda/pop), crisps (potato chips) have lots of carbohydrates and are high GI.

- If meals are missed or not enough is eaten, then the blood glucose will drop too low, you may become hypoglycaemic from the low blood glucose which can cause sudden confusion (delirium), but it is commonly unrecognised by the elderly. If you already have dementia then a low blood glucose (hypoglycaemic episode) can worsen your dementia. If you have a balance or walking problem it can make that worse too.

- Low GI foods do not cause a spike in blood glucose and are better for elderly diabetics.

## GOOD CARBOHYDRATE FOODS FOR ELDERLY DIABETICS:

- Oats, porridge, pasta, rice and crackers.

- Vegetables– such as sweet potatoes, corn.

- Dairy products -milk, yoghurt, custard.

- Fruit- oranges, bananas, apples.

- Legumes (these are Split peas, Kidney beans, Cannellini beans, Soy Beans, Baked beans, Four bean mix, red, green, brown Lentils) – these are good for diabetics because they are high in fibre so good for bowels, good source of protein and carbohydrate.

## CAN ELDERLY DIABETICS EAT SUGAR?

A small amount of sugar is OK in coffee, tea, or on cereal, and honey or jam on bread.

Diabetics should avoid high GI foods that are high in sugar such as soft drinks (soda/pop), cordial, juices, jelly, chocolates, sweet biscuits and cakes, as these will elevate the blood glucose and make diabetic control difficult. When diabetes is being assessed or needing to be stabilised, the older person should avoid very high GI foods which may give the Doctor a false impression of poor diabetic control and over-treat them. This may cause the Doctor to increase the oral diabetic pills or the Insulin dose and then when sugar intake is reduced in the diet, the older diabetic will end up with a hypoglycaemic episode.

# SWALLOWING DIFFICULTIES

Most older people can swallow solids and liquids normally, however swallowing impairments and incoordinated swallows are increasingly common in frail older people, particularly with neurological impairments such as Parkinson's, stroke and dementia. These types of patients can lose the co-ordination in swallowing and something that we take for granted can become a major issue for them.

Regular coughing after swallowing liquids or solids is a sign of swallowing dyspraxia (incoordinated swallow) and a risk for silent aspiration (food or fluid going down the wrong way into the lungs) contributing to recurrent chest infections and potentially fatal pneumonia. . Swallowing difficulties commonly cause a chronic rattly cough. They also have difficulty swallowing pills which may be the first sign of swallowing dyspraxia.

These patients should be appropriately assessed by a Speech Pathologist in terms of the correct food and fluid consistency, the best head position when swallowing and other exercises to reduce the risk of it going down the wrong way.

- The best head position is sitting upright and forward to reduce the risk of silent aspiration and the food or fluid going down the wrong way.
- Slouching back in a lounge chair or bed is the worst position when eating and drinking for a frail older person.
- They may require a sip of fluid with each swallow of solid food to help it go down.
- They should avoid distraction.

- They should have good oral hygiene and appropriate mouth care to keep their mouth clean and moist.
- They sometimes require altered textured food including cut up food with gravy to assist in swallowing and sometimes thickened fluid which is easy to swallow when the swallowing co-ordination is impaired. Those elderly patients on thickened fluids need to be monitored carefully for dehydration, as older patients do not like thickened fluids and tend to restrict their fluid intake when on them. We always have to balance comfort and quality of life versus the risk of silent aspiration and pneumonia in these types of patients.
- They may need to swallow their pills with custard or yoghurt which improves the swallowing coordination.

Other causes for impaired swallowing include:

- Sedative and anti-psychotic medications which can make the patient drowsy and confused and make the incoordination of swallowing worse.
- Drugs that can dry out the mouth including anti-cholinergic type drugs.

Swallowing should always be assessed in patients with delirium, dementia, falls or in the post-operative period after a general anaesthetic which can increase the risk of delirium and post-operative cognitive decline.

## THE GAMA SYNDROME

This impairment of swallowing which I have named GAMA syndrome (unpublished) occurs in frail older people with-
- G-poor walking balance (gait ataxia).
- A-Alzheimer's Dementia.
- M-Malnutrition.
- A-Silent aspiration of food and fluids.

I have seen this so many times in my medical practice over many years. These people commonly have unrecognised weak and incoordinated swallowing. This causes food and liquids to go down the wrong way into their lungs, thus increasing their risk for recurrent chest infections and pneumonia. It is very common in such frail people because they have an underlying neuro-degenerative brain disorder affecting their balance and swallowing. They are commonly malnourished because they cannot eat enough due to their swallowing impairment and have reduced appetite from dementia. These type of patients should always have their swallowing assessed.

# ADVERSE DRUG REACTIONS/DRUG SIDE EFFECTS

Adverse drug reactions are very common in the elderly but most are predictable and preventable!

The elderly are the greatest consumers of medications. They have the greatest number of side effects. Drug side effects are much more common in people over 65 years of age and older. They are associated with a higher risk of serious complications and death. They are the most significant treatable, preventable "health problem" in older people and contribute to avoidable hospital Emergency Department presentations.

Older people with drug side effects tend to present differently with confusion, falls, immobility and incontinence, as compared to younger patients.

Drug interactions are very common, but are under-recognised and undertreated in the elderly.

Risk factors for adverse drug reactions in the elderly-
- Inappropriate prescribing is common in the elderly due to multiple presentations to multiple single organ Doctors (SODs) where everyone is adding their little bit of medication, but there is no-one overall coordinating the treatment.

- Poor geriatric prescribing knowledge and lack of awareness of how the elderly body handles the medications.

- Glossy advertisements with little data specific for the elderly, with many drugs specifically studied in younger, fitter, paid volunteers, with minimal data extrapolated for marketing for the elderly.

- The elderly have impaired reserve to tolerate larger doses of drugs.

- The most important risk factor for adverse drug reactions is the number of drugs taken.

90% of adverse drug reactions in the elderly are preventable. They result in a 7 times risk of hospital Emergency department presentation versus younger people.

People over 65 years of age comprise about 12% of the population, but account for about 66% of prescribed medications.

While there are a few more drug studies including people over the age of 80 years, there are limitations in our ability to extrapolate and predict the results of therapeutic drug trials to older patients we see in daily practice.

Many drug trials specifically exclude older individuals such as those over 80 years or those with frailty and multiple co-morbidities because it is just too hard and too complex to administer the studies.

About 1 in 4 older people take at least 5 prescribed medications. Published data suggest that over 30% of hospital admissions for the elderly are due to adverse drug reactions. Up to 80% are preventable.

The therapeutic window of drug benefit versus toxic drug side effects narrows as we get older, and is predictable as the drug doses increase.

Older people are more prone to Type A adverse drug reactions which are dose related, predictable, and related to the pharmacological actions of the drug. Type B adverse drug reactions are usually uncommon and unrelated to the pharmacological reactions of the drug or doses and are quite unpredictable, including rashes and low blood counts or low serum sodium (hyponatraemia).

Randomised drug trials are seldom designed to detect increases in falls, functional impairment and cognitive impairment which are amongst the most common adverse drug events in older adults.

Protocol driven medicine based on flawed published studies which never include the frail elderly patients that I see, and fail to publish side effects of treatments such as low standing blood pressures and falls contribute to more drug side effects and poorer health outcomes. Treatments for the elderly must be based on individual patients needs and taking into account risks of standard drug doses. Evidence-based medicine must include the frail elderly in studies to allow Doctors to make the safest and most effective treatment choices.

There is a clear association between the number of falls and the types and number of medications used in the elderly.

Exposure to any psychotropic medication, regardless of class, is associated with almost a two-fold increase in falls in older adults.

Newer psychotropic medications such as atypical anti-psychotics have been associated with a similar falls risk in older adults compared to the older psychotropic type drugs. There is a clear association between falls risk and sedative anti-psychotics medication with the elderly.

Medication side effects have been reported to be the cause of 25% of cases of in-hospital delirium.

Drug classes most strongly associated with cognitive impairment and delirium are psychotropic and anti-cholinergic medications. Parkinson's Disease drugs can also cause confusion and hallucinations.

Malnourished elderly have a much higher risk of adverse drug reactions because they have a decreased body mass and muscle mass is a good sump for absorbing drugs to prevent side effects. There is decreased serum albumin (protein in the circulation) to bind the free drug.

Elderly people are commonly dehydrated, so they have a higher peak serum concentration of the drugs targeting organs such as the brain, the heart, the liver and the kidneys. They commonly have multiple chronic disease processes which make them more vulnerable to adverse drug reactions.

Adverse drug reactions are commonly missed and more importantly, drug interactions or drug to drug effects are even more commonly missed. There is the potential for major drug interactions with complementary or herbal therapies, along with traditional medications. There is also the concern of elderly people taking self-prescribed over the counter medications, causing further drug interactions.

I like the use of medication packs which are made up by the Chemist and the patient given a 7 day supply. It is sealed and is easily visible. The medications are clearly listed and if the doses are missed the window is still there showing the medications that were missed.

For one of my studies on elderly patients with adverse drug reactions presenting to the hospital emergency department, I had found that of the 267 geriatric patients presenting-

- the average number of medications taken were 6.2 per patient.
- The percentage of adverse drug reactions was 50%, directly contributing to the Emergency Department presentation.
- Drug interactions were about 12%.
- Good drug compliance about 70%.
- Medication was supervised by others in at least 60% of patients.
- Over 80% of patients presented with major geriatric syndromes as a result of adverse drug reactions.
- Only about 19% were able to name their medications accurately.

## POOR MEDICATION KNOWLEGE

I commonly see patients in my rooms who do not bring their medications with them and have no idea what they are taking. They are unable to tell me the names of the medications, the doses or strengths of the pills, the frequency of administration, the reason for taking the medications and any knowledge of potential adverse drug reactions. They commonly say "No one asked me to bring my pills" when we have already told them to do so! Reviewing medications with each Doctor appointment is so important. It's a bit like not bringing your car when booked in for a car service! People expect top medical care, yet how can the Doctor safely prescribe new medication without accurately knowing what the patient is already taking? When I ask them for the names of all of their pills, they commonly say "yes, of course I can name my pills"! but then go on to say the blue pill and the white one", they say mls (millilitres) which means liquid volume rather than mg (milligrams) which refers to drug strength and just have no idea about what they are taking! This commonly indicates underlying cognitive impairment/dementia. If you can't name your pills and doses accurately then you need a pill pack made up by the chemist. Poor medication knowledge by older patients contributes to adverse drug reactions.

Many of these older patients also love to fiddle with their pills when they can't name any of them and put them into a dosette box which increases the risk of medication errors by excess handling of multiple pills.

## ALTERED DRUG METABOLISM IN THE ELDERLY

The older body does handle drugs differently to a younger person. There is a decline in body size. There is a decline in total body water so that drug concentrations are higher. There is a decline in lean body muscle mass, so that there is less muscle to absorb excess drugs. There is a decline in liver mass, so the liver is less able to metabolise the drugs, along with a decrease in liver blood flow to extract drugs from the system. There is a decline in renal function, reducing the ability of the body to excrete the drugs.

Nevertheless, if appropriately prescribed and the dose calculated for age and renal function, you can minimise the risk of adverse drug reactions in the elderly.

Renal function declines every decade after the age of 60. But that does not mean you develop renal (kidney) failure just because you are old. It just means that the older kidney has less reserve to cope with any stress such as dehydration, infections and drug side effects. Drug doses should be calculated by body weight and by serum Creatinine which is a measure of renal function, to get the correct dose and reduce adverse drug reactions.

Certain drugs can have the blood levels monitored to prevent adverse drug reactions including anti-epileptic drugs, Lithium and Digoxin for the heart.

We weigh neonates (new born babies) and children to calculate safe drug doses for low body weight, but older patients are not routinely weighed to calculate their drug doses to reduce the number of adverse drug reactions. Nor are elderly patients' nutritional states routinely screened and assessed for malnutrition when this also can have a huge impact on adverse drug reactions.

## ANTI-COAGULANTS

Anti-coagulants or blood thinners are being prescribed much more frequently in elderly patients now. Drugs such as Warfarin and NOAC (Novel) anti-coagulants have been shown to significantly reduce the risk of stroke with AF (irregular heart rhythm) by about two thirds. This is when the heart can throw off a clot to the brain. However the bleeding risk also significantly increases in the older patient. The NOACs are not reversible like Warfarin can be with Vit K. Patients on anti-coagulants should avoid NSAIDs arthritis drugs such as Ibuprofen due to the increased risk of bleeding from the stomach. Those patients who are also on Aspirin for coronary stents have a higher risk of severe anaemia so must be monitored carefully. There is an increased risk of drug interactions and bleeding risk with anti-coagulants and other drugs including herbals and "complimentary medicines".

The question posed today about anti-coagulants though is, not why should we use them for the older patient, but why shouldn't we use them? The stroke risk reduction with AF is significant and those with increased risk factors for AF stroke have the most to benefit such as those with:

- Hypertension
- Heart failure
- Previous stroke/TIA
- Vascular disease
- Diabetes
- Over 75 years of age

Aspirin is still used too much and should be reserved for secondary stoke prevention, coronary artery disease and coronary artery stents or vascular stents. Just using low dose Aspirin alone as a blood thinner for "preventative medicine" in the otherwise well elderly has been shown to be harmful and can shorten life and increase bleeding risk. It has a higher risk of major haemorrhage and does not reduce cardiovascular disease in the elderly.

## COMMON CLASSESS OF DRUGS CAUSING ADVERSE DRUG REACTIONS IN THE ELDERLY:

- Blood pressure pills causing postural hypotension and falls.
- Heart failure pills causing postural hypotension and falls.
- Diuretics causing dehydration, kidney failure, low serum potassium and sodium.
- Anti-psychotics causing worsening balance, falls, confusion.

- Tricyclic anti-depressants causing postural hypotension, dry eyes, dry mouth, constipation, falls, confusion, worsening heart failure.
- NSAIDs (non-steroidal anti-inflammatory) drugs for arthritis causing gastro-intestinal bleeding and kidney failure and high serum potassium.
- Anti-coagulants causing bleeding in bowels, brain, kidney, skin.
- Steroids like Prednisone causing osteoporosis, high blood glucose, leg swelling, muscle weakness, skin bruising.
- Oral hypoglycaemic diabetic pills causing prolonged low blood glucose (hypos) confusion and falls.
- Narcotic analgesia causing nausea, drowsiness, constipation, confusion, falls.
- Nerve pain pills (Gabapentin, Pregabalin) causing drowsiness, falls, confusion.
- Diazepam and other sedatives/sleeping pills causing falls, confusion, worsening incontinence, worsening swallowing.

Several years ago I calculated the cost of preventable acute hospital admissions for the elderly with adverse drug reactions.
- The average length of hospital stay was 10 days
- Cost was $1000 per day or $10,000 per admission.
- Give 50% of all elderly admissions to hospital may be due to adverse drug reactions this is a huge avoidable cost to State and Federal Government health departments!

## HOW TO AVOID ADVERSE DRUG REACTIONS IN THE ELDERLY:

- Is the indication for the medication still present?

- Is the disease modifying treatment still helping symptoms?
- Is there an acceptable balance between efficacy and adverse effects?
- Is the dose appropriate for the older frailer patient?
- Are there any potential drug interactions?
- Are there better alternatives, either pharmacological or non-pharmacological?
- Weigh the patient.
- Calculate drug doses for age, weight, kidney function.
- Take into account other disease present such as chronic heart, lung, kidney, and liver disease which may mean reducing drug doses to avoid side effects.
- Educate the patient, family and Carers all about the drug doses, actions and possible side effects.
- Monitor for adverse drug reactions and drug to drug interactions.
- Use pill packs delivered by the local Chemist to improve drug compliance when on multiple pills.

## BEST TREATMENT FOR DEPRESSION IN THE ELDERLY

The best treatment for depression, worry, low mood and despair in the elderly is not more drugs but the Wests Tigers Rugby League jersey. When I wear this bright colourful white, orange and black striped jersey with a Tiger emblem on my hospital ward rounds on casual days, it immediately brightens up the mood and wakes up lethargic and unwell elderly patients who just love the bright colours and positive vibe it produces. It works every time and guess what- no side effects! It even helps patients with dementia who start interacting better with staff when they see the Wests Tigers Jersey. All staff should be wearing a colourful uniform, and if I had my way, all Doctors, nurses, and other staff should all be wearing the Wests Tigers Rugby league jersey!

Yes, anti-depressant medications have a proven role in treatment of severe depression in the elderly, but they can have significant side effects. Non-drug strategies should always be tried first. However, older people with severe depression tend to get the physical symptoms more commonly such as loss of appetite, weight loss, insomnia, lethargy, slowing up generally, constipation, agitation more than the cognitive or emotional symptoms such as depressed mood, loss of interest and enjoyment in things, feeling helpless, excessive worry, feeling worthlessness, irritability, loss of energy, feeling excessively tired, concentration problems, and recurrent thoughts of death. These people generally require anti-depressant medication.

# SLEEPING PILLS

Don't take sleeping pills! That's the simple answer! The Benzodiazepine class of sleeping pills have serious side effects in the elderly. Benzodiazepine sleeping pills include Temazepam, Oxazepam, Diazepam, and other classes include Amitriptyline (tricyclic anti-depressants), Doxylamine (sedating anti-histamine), Zolpidem, Zopiclone. Many older ladies complain bitterly that they can't sleep but observations in hospital show that most do sleep but still complain about insomnia. Sleeping pills are addictive and levels build up in the body. Even the so-called shorter acting sleeping pills such as Temazepam and Oxazepam build up levels in the blood so that the body never fully gets rid of the drug before the next dose. Older people are then permanently "drugged up to their eye balls and "zonked" all day. Even when long-acting Benzodiazepines such as Diazepam are stopped, the drug and its sedative effects may persist in the body for more than 2 weeks later! Increased falls risk is no different between the shorter acting and longer acting sleeping pills. Even narcotic pain killers can affect sleep and cause awakenings even though they are sedative drugs. Most of these sleeping pills are shockers because they have so many side effects with very little or no benefit!

Causes for insomnia include-

- Breathlessness from untreated heart failure.
- Gastro-oesophageal reflux causing recurrent coughing at night.
- Leg and foot cramps.
- Painful osteoarthritis in hips and knees.

- Restless legs.
- Rapid eye movement (REM) sleep behaviour disorder.
- Nocturia- frequently getting up to go to the toilet to pass urine.
- Restlessness complicating Dementia.
- Too many day-time naps.
- Obstructive sleep apnoea.

Side effects of sleeping pills include:

- Confusion.
- Worsening balance and falls.
- Swallowing impairment.
- Incontinence.
- Next daytime drowsiness.
- Physical and psychological addiction.

Suddenly stopping sleeping pills that a person has been taking for years can cause rapid withdrawal symptoms such as worsening insomnia, agitation, confusion (delirium), falls and even seizures. These sleeping pills must be gradually withdrawn and tapered under close medical supervision to avoid serious withdrawal complications.

## INSOMNIA IN THE ELDERLY

Chronic insomnia affects about 20% of the elderly. Most sleep OK. Sleep generally becomes lighter, shorter duration, and more fragmented in some older people. There are more awakenings during the night. Ageing can be associated with a decrease in sleep quality. This is caused by lowered melatonin levels, altered circadian rhythms, and multiple medical co-morbidities (other illnesses). Older people can have delayed sleep onset, and more daytime sleepiness/tiredness as a result of poor sleep. Deep stage 4 sleep is important for good health. It allows the body to "recover", it stabilises metabolism, and consolidates memories. REM sleep comes in 90 minute cycles. The percentage of time spent in REM sleep decreases with age. Circadian rhythm (healthy 24 hour body clock) disturbances are more severe and more disabling in people with dementia compared with healthy older adults. Dementia patients have frequent awakenings at night, restlessness and wandering. They commonly have altered day/night awareness, so they may get dressed to go to work at 2am or want breakfast at midnight. Parkinson's disease patients frequently have sleep disturbances due to the Parkinson's disease tremor, rigidity, restlessness and overactive bladder. They may also get nocturnal confusion, agitation, hallucinations from side effects of their Parkinson's medications. These symptoms are all treatable!

## REM SLEEP BEHAVIOUR DISORDER

Normal REM sleep allows the body to lay down memories, consolidate emotions and dreams, but the muscles are paralysed during REM sleep to prevent the dreams being acted out. REM sleep behaviour disorders (RBD) in the elderly can cause the person to act out dreams that emerge during a loss of REM sleep so that they may start kicking, punching, and thrashing around in bed. They can injure their partner in bed. RBD can be caused by anti-depressant medications. RBD can also be caused by the brain syndrome of alpha-synuclein neurodegeneration. This is a warning sign of increased risk for developing Parkinson's disease and other similar neurodegenerative disorders such as dementia with Lewy Bodies, and multi-system brain atrophy. Melatonin tablets may help RBD. It tends to be better tolerated than the more sedating alternative  Clonazepam tablets but this can work better in older adults with neurodegenerative disorders.

## BENZODIAZEPINE SLEEPING PILLS

Long-acting Benzodiazepines sleeping pills such as Diazepam are associated with mild improvements in sleep duration, but they suppress deep sleep which impairs the sleep's restorative effects. Benefits associated with sedative pills are outweighed by the risk of adverse drug side effects, particularly those frail elderly at a high risk for confusion and falls. Older people have increased sensitivity to drug side effects despite growing tolerance to the sedative effects. Side effects include daytime drowsiness, fatigue, lethargy, loss of energy, loss of "drive and get-up and go", depression, memory loss, paradoxical agitation, impaired coordination and falls. Benzodiazepines and other sleeping pills may also worsen cognitive decline in people who already have dementia. They can worsen swallowing coordination and cause or worsen incontinence. They suppress (REM) sleep which is known to have a role in learning and memory consolidation, so may increase risk for confusion. Shorter acting sleeping pills such as Temazepam and Oxazepam can worsen night time sleep quality and cause longer day time napping. These sleeping pills can cause memory impairment. All sleeping pills can cause respiratory depression in those with chronic lung disease. With prolonged use these sleeping pills lose their sleep producing effects. The body just gets used to them. Older people then become addicted to them like drug addicts!

## CRAMPS

Leg cramps at night are a common cause of insomnia and poor sleep. Cramps may be due to poor circulation, peripheral neuropathy or abnormal serum electrolytes such as low magnesium or calcium. A proper medical diagnosis is needed first. Magnesium tablets may help. Another simple remedy is a small glass of Indian Tonic Water which contains quinine which helps leg cramps.

## RESTLESS LEGS

Restless legs at night are a common cause of poor fragmented sleep. It is characterised by an uncomfortable feeling of constant leg movements, jerking and restlessness almost like riding a bike or walking in bed. It can last for hours. It causes daytime tiredness due to night time sleep interruption. Treatment includes low does Levodopa which is used in Parkinson's disease or Pramipexole tablets.

Periodic limb movements or nocturnal myoclonus, and jerky involuntary movements of the legs during sleep lasting up to 10 seconds at a time but are not associated with painful leg cramps. It can be diagnosed on a formal sleep study.

Nocturnal myoclonus is the sudden, short, jerky or shock-like, involuntary movements caused by muscular contractions of arms or legs. It can result in injury to the partner in bed. Drugs such as Clonazepam or anti-epileptics such as Valproate may help.

# MALNUTRITION IN THE ELDERLY

You do not become malnourished and lose weight because you are old!

Malnutrition in the elderly is one of the greatest challenges facing the health system. It is a very common problem but potentially treatable and reversible. It contributes to serious complications and early death in the elderly.

Over 50% of acute geriatric medical hospitalised patients and nursing home patients have some form of significant malnutrition. The prevalence of this problem in community living elderly over 65 years of age is at least 30%.

Malnutrition in older people is clearly associated with-
* increased complications and death rate.
* increased risk for infection and falls.
* longer and more complicated and expensive hospital stay.

These are potentially treatable/preventable.

Older people at particular risk of malnutrition include those with-
* Alzheimer's dementia.
* Parkinson's disease.
* stroke.
* fractured hip.
* chronic lung disease.
* heart failure.
* the disabled housebound older person.
* those with chewing and swallowing problems.

Malnutrition in the elderly is commonly associated with multiple chronic medical problems, leading to an early and unnecessary preventable hospital admission. Malnourished elderly are simply not consuming enough calories and protein to meet their metabolic demands to maintain their weight and bodily function.

Malnutrition in the elderly is commonly associated with-
- muscle weakness and wasting,
- deteriorating mobility,
- ankle swelling,
- dehydration,
- confusion,
- falls,
- impaired immune function, so that they are less able to fight infections,
- alters the way the body handles medication resulting in increased concentration of drugs in the body and increases the risk of adverse drug reactions.

Studies have shown that geriatric malnutrition is commonly ignored and under-recognised in the acute and chronic hospital setting.

Routine regular screening tools for malnutrition are essential in identifying high risk patients from malnutrition. This will enable early intervention and appropriate treatment to prevent the complications of malnutrition.

## ENFORCED STARVATION OF THE ELDERLY

Many older patients have dyspraxia or poor co-ordination with swallowing, with silent aspiration (food and fluid going down the wrong way) and are very slow eaters which is common but under-recognised. Food services in Residential Aged Care and acute hospital settings need to target these older people at risk of malnutrition and provide appropriate food consistencies, enough time to consume the meals, correct positioning for meals, preferably out of bed, sitting upright to reduce the risk of choking or silent aspiration and feeding assistance as required. Food packaging is so difficult to open, you almost need a jack-hammer to open the butter, jam, biscuits, and juice packets. More than half the frail elderly patients in hospital need assistance with meals and opening food packets, and most in aged care hostels and nursing homes need assistance with meals. More than half of the older patients in hospital are very slow eaters and can take over 1 hour to eat a meal. Unfortunately, quite commonly food delivery services put a time limit on how long they will leave the meal trays out with patients and then efficiently and abruptly remove the trays from the frail and disabled elderly patients before they have had time to consume all of their meal. This is a result of the hospital or the institution prioritising food service staff work time and shifts, as opposed to patient's needs for better nutrition, lack of observation, monitoring and reporting of uneaten meals to send a warning sign out that the patient needs to be assessed as to why they are not eating. Lack of nutritional assessment and monitoring enforces starvation within the hospital, and in the Residential Aged Care setting.

All food services staff who assist in meal menu selection and deliver meals to frail elderly patients in hospitals must have some form of training in recognising confusion, swallowing difficulties, malnutrition and feeding assistance. I published a study on this very topic highlighting the need to monitor the amount of food older patients in hospital have left uneaten for each meal and report that in the medical records for further assessment and management. Undereating must NOT be ignored as it usually is in hospitals! I developed a system of a BLUE place mat on the meal tray for those who require altered texture meals and fluids due to swallowing difficulties and needing extra monitoring by nursing staff, and a RED place mat for those frail elderly patients who require hand-on feeding assistance. ("Improving Food Delivery Services for Acute Hospital Geriatric Inpatients". A quality assurance project. (Poster presentation for The Australian Society for Geriatric Medicine Annual Scientific Meeting, Cairns, July 2000).

I also published several papers on malnutrition in the elderly which generated significant newspaper, TV and radio headlines such as "Elderly Starved of Nutrition in Homes" and "Fed or Dead". Governments don't like these headlines. Unfortunately little has changed with the nutritional care of the elderly since.

Malnutrition is such a common problem leading to potentially catastrophic complications and outcomes, yet it is easily fixed but is still commonly ignored.

## POOR ATTITUDE TO HOSPITAL FOOD

Most hospitals relegate nutritional services to the hotel or "basement" services and minimise resourcing for Dietitians. We spend millions of dollars on unnecessary medical investigations, and on toxic medications, but we spend absolutely the minimum on food services and nutrition. This is a paradox, as for every dollar that is spent on improving nutrition and food delivery services, $10 is saved for Governments in health costs in the acute hospital setting.

Many hospitals try to save money by spending at little as possible on food. This just doesn't make sense! This is anti-patient, anti-science and just plain stupid! Good food is essential for healing and is a super medicine for frail older patients. Who wouldn't want to save Grandma or Grandad by providing high quality nutritious food? Food heals and food is health. You are what you eat! Hospital food should be gourmet and not the cheapest lowest common denominator of frozen over cooked tasteless meals with all of the vitamins and other nutrients cooked out, but rather serving fresh linguine with pan fried salmon in olive oil packed with Omega 3 oils and fresh colourful vegetables. Even soft and puree meals can be nutritious and presented attractively rather than just slop!

Many high quality fresh foods have health benefits. Lycopenes are plant nutrients with antioxidant benefits. They are super foods such as tomatoes and watermelons. Lycopenes may protect against cancer and heart disease and improve cholesterol levels. Phytochemicals in fruit and vegetables add to super food health benefits. These include Carotenoids in carrots and broccoli, with benefits in reducing cancer and cardiovascular disease, Flavonoids in berries, apples, onions help fight inflammation, Resveratrol in grapes, dark chocolate and Anthocyanins in berries all have health benefits.

It is quite amazing that such crazy decisions made by unqualified people running hospitals to starve patients by spending as little as possible on food and nutrition services still go on despite the scientific evidence that better nutrition improves health outcomes, and that malnutrition results in longer length of hospital stay, more complications, and much higher health care costs. Who are these hospital managers? We wouldn't let the passenger fly the plane so why are critical decisions in hospital management made by unqualified people? We need to have the debate- should hospitals be run by Doctors or non-medical managers? This also brings up the bigger issue of politics. Health is so important that should we allow a Local Member of Parliament to become the Health Minister to make critical decisions about our health when they have no medical qualifications. What medical qualifications does the Health Minister's Chief of Staff or Principal Private Secretary have? Who is advising the Health Minister, then who is advising the Minister's advisers? Health expertise needs to be portfolio specific with a qualified Doctor running it. My model would be no unqualified Health Minister, but rather a committee of a Physician, a Surgeon and a Nurse running health and reporting directly to the State Premier or State Governor.

All older people should undergo some form of nutritional assessment, whether they are in the hospital Emergency Department, acute hospital, Doctor's Surgery or in Residential Aged Care.

Simple high calorie protein drink supplements have been shown to reduce the complications of protein energy malnutrition.

A multi-disciplinary approach to nutritional support should be promoted involving speech pathologist, nutritionist and holistic medical care, with early mobility (improving their walking and balance).

Improving the nutritional status of older people should be promoted as a very high priority health strategy.

# COMPLICATIONS OF MALNUTRITION

- Worsens the outcome of chronic illness.
- Worsens the outcome of post-operative surgical patients, and particularly fractured neck of femur patients.
- Increases the risk of infections, falls and delirium.
- Decreases muscle strength.
- Poor wound healing.

One of my previous published statements was "It is quite a paradox of modern medicine that most Doctors pay little attention to the nutritional status of the elderly when it is such a common problem, leading to potentially catastrophic outcomes, yet is potentially reversible" - Lipski 1997.

Older people with dementia living alone have a high risk of malnutrition. They tend to restrict the amount of calories and protein they eat, but this can improve with company when family visit or when they go out.

Frail elderly generally eat mostly food of a low nutrient density.

At times of high energy requirements such as during body stress with an acute on chronic illness, they don't get enough calories or protein which results in a deficit and malnutrition.

Elderly people rapidly become "hypercatabolic" with an increase in their metabolic rate and energy requirements during periods of infection and acute illness. Then they develop rapid muscle weakness and wasting and a cascade of malnutrition complications including the dreaded ankle swelling and immobility.

Multivitamins alone have no value in malnutrition, as these patients are deficient in calories and protein.

The taste sensation diminishes in the elderly, so food flavours, enhancers and sometimes salt can be beneficial in improving appetite.

Poor dentition and oral hygiene also contribute to impaired swallowing and reduced food intake.

## PROTEIN ENERGY MALNUTRITION

This is a metabolic response to stress in an older person's body that results in a significant increase in protein and energy requirements to maintain balance. Inadequate nutrient supply then affects organ systems within as little time as 2-3 days of inadequate intake. Acute confusion/delirium is often seen in protein energy malnutrition and related to dehydration as well.

## MULTIFACTORIAL NATURE OF MALNUTRITION IN THE ELDERLY

This is not just attributed to poor intake alone. Many drugs can cause nausea, impair appetite, dry mouth and impair swallowing.

The average dietary requirement for younger fitter people is about 8500kJ per day. About 55% of your daily energy (kilojoules) will come from carbohydrates and sugary foods.

The carbohydrates in the elderly are essential to prevent the body breaking down fat and muscle to make glucose for the brain and other organs.

In terms of protein, the requirements can be up to 25% of your energy or at least 1g/kg of ideal body weight per day, probably more in the frail elderly. Protein supplements in the frail malnourished elderly help to build up muscle.

The rest of the kilojoules, about 20% comes from fat. Again, this is a good source of calories for frail older people.

## "MAKING EVERY MOUTHFUL COUNT":

This is an important concept of getting an older frail person to eat more calories/kilojoules and protein in every mouthful by better selection of foods, fortifying meals and have more frequent snacks.

## WARNING SIGNS OF MALNUTRITION:

- Loss of appetite.
- Losing interest in food.
- Losing weight
- Having smaller meals than usual.
- Having fewer snacks.
- Missing meals.
- Chronic nausea.
- Swallowing problems.
- Teeth and mouth problems.
- Chronic pain.
- Depression.
- Confusion.
- Excess alcohol consumption.
- Social isolation.
- Walking and balance problems.

This is not a part of "normal ageing". Rather, these are warning signs that the elderly person needs more calories/kilojoules and protein in their diet just to stay healthy and avoid muscle breakdown and weight loss.

## **HOW TO IMPROVE FOOD INTAKE AND APPETITE:**

- Eat smaller more frequent meals. Try 5-6 smaller meals a day rather than the traditional 3 large meals. Larger meals may "put off" the older person with an already poor appetite.

- Have small plates so meals appear smaller and more tempting than larger ones.

- Have scrambled eggs or porridge with cream any time of the day like a snack, not just for breakfast.

- Have some high calorie snacks between meals such as chocolate biscuits, cakes, full cream yoghurt, cream caramel, crisps (potato chips) for extra calories.

- Avoid bland salads, plain dry biscuits and low fat foods which do not have enough calories (energy) and protein which the older person needs.

## **ENERGY FOODS-KILOJOULES:**

- Energy foods (calories or kilojoules) are essential to prevent muscle breakdown and weight loss. They may also improve appetite, particularly in those with nausea.

- Don't have low fat dairy products. Avoid low fat milk! It doesn't have enough energy and food value in it!

- High energy snacks include full cream milk and yoghurt, butter, margarine, ice cream, soft drinks (pop/soda), chocolates, sweet biscuits, ice cream, cakes, meat pies, sausage rolls and chips.

- Add 2 heaped tablespoons of full sour cream in soups, grated cheese on food, use thick butter on vegetables.

## PROTEIN:

- Frail, complex older patients need more protein just to maintain weight and prevent muscle breakdown. To get enough protein older people need have some at every meal.

- Eggs are really the best source of protein as they are easily digestible, easy to prepare and tasty.

- I recommend as least 3 scrambled eggs for breakfast or lunch with thick butter spread on 2 slices of toast.

- High protein foods include red meat, pork, fish, chicken, eggs, legumes, beans. Also dairy products such as full cream milk and yoghurt, cheese.

## NUTRITIONAL SUPPLEMENTS:

Commercial high protein energy fortified supplements may also be needed in those elderly who are simply still not eating enough to meet their metabolic nutritional demands. . These can be either a high protein energy milk drink or pudding snack in between meals 3 times a day. High energy protein powder, at least 2 heaped tablespoons can be sprinkled on breakfast cereal and porridge, custards, desserts, soups, even on cooked food, or made up into drinks to add extra nutrients and energy to food.

## MULTI-VITAMINS

Many older people love to take multi-vitamins but they have no proof in preventing major Geriatric Syndromes such as confusion, falls and malnutrition. Vitamins do not have calories or protein so do not improve malnutrition. Older people commonly take many multi-vitamins and complementary medicines just to stay "healthy" with significant cost but there is no proven value here, particularly when their diet is inadequate. They may also interact with other medications. I have never seen complimentary medicines improve memory loss or reduce the risk of dementia. Anti-oxidants such as Vitamin A, E, and beta carotene can increase cancer risk and mortality when taken in excess. They are found in fruits, berries and veggies, so eat them instead. Selenium can increase cancer risk in high doses. Vit C does not prevent viral illness in older people but can increase the risk of kidney stones in high doses. But yes, I do recommend multi-vitamins for malnutrition but only in combination with high protein high energy diets. If the older person ate proper food and enough of it in the first place, then they wouldn't need to spend money on multi-vitamins! I also use Thiamine Vitamin B1 tabs for severe malnutrition to prevent the re-feeding syndrome when the frail elderly person starts eating properly again. Thiamine protects the brain from nutritional encephalopathy (acute confusion) and body electrolyte disturbances (low serum potassium, magnesium and phosphate) during re-feeding. Older people tend not to eat enough foods containing Thiamine such as bread, cereals, and pasta. Overall though, multi-vitamins are not a substitute for poor eating.

## SALADS AND "CARDBOARD" BREAKFAST-

I usually get the same reaction from both the patient and the relatives who generally sit back in their chair, their eyes roll back and they appear most surprised that I am saying to them to eat 2 or 3 times what they are currently eating, just to maintain their health and weight.

The misconception in the community is that as you get older you eat less is so ingrained that it takes a lot of effort to convince people otherwise that without significantly improving calorie and protein intake in older people, they will suffer the serious consequences of malnutrition.

While the "Dr Lipski diet" of cakes, sweets, chocolate biscuits, ice cream, custards, meat pies, sausage rolls and hamburgers may be very suitable for frail malnourished elderly, they are not necessary for otherwise fit and healthy elderly.

Many older people are still obsessed with eating low fat foods such as skim milk, having too many salads without protein, and bland "cardboard" breakfast cereal without calories. There is really no role for low fat milk or other low fat dairy products in older frail people. The risks of malnutrition far outweigh any concern about higher cholesterol level here. Salads and "cardboard" breakfast cereals simply do not offer enough calories or protein to sustain health and body weight in frail elderly. They should at least be adding to their salads eggs, cheese and meat on top. The best breakfast for frail elderly is of course 3 scrambled eggs and bacon on toast with thick butter!

## DON'T LOSE WEIGHT AS YOU GET OLDER!

As you get older you should NOT try to lose weight unless you have morbid obesity. I still see many older women who are obsessed about losing weight, staying thin, and dieting when it is unnecessary and potentially dangerous to their health. These older women tend to eat very low energy foods such as salads and very small portions only, thus putting themselves at risk of malnutrition and its complications. Older people need to have some reserve in body weight when they become ill. Older people can rapidly lose weight during periods of acute illness such as infections, inflammation, falls and subsequent immobility. These adverse events produce extra stress on the body, so demands for energy and protein go up.

If the older person is not eating enough kilojoules and protein, then they burn up body fat to make energy. If they are too skinny/underweight with very little body fat, then their muscles rapidly break down to make glucose for the brain and other vital organs. The liver then cannot keep up making protein for the body, ankle swelling starts, as protein (albumin) drops in the circulation. The circulating protein usually helps to keep fluid from leaking out of the legs and ankles. When the older person becomes malnourished, they also become immuno-suppressed. They then cannot fight infections well, so more easily develop serious infections and complications such as delirium, falls and pressure ulcers on their heels and sacrum and paper thin skin.

## MY MOTHER IS OLD SO SHE DOESN'T NEED TO EAT MUCH YOU KNOW!

How often do I hear this! "You know Doctor, my Mother is 85 years old now". "You know she doesn't do much so she doesn't need to eat much".
How wrong can you be!!
This myth about frail older people needing to eat less is such a widely held belief among families.
There is no science behind it. In fact, if the older person is frail, with multiple chronic medical conditions, and poor mobility with muscle weakness, then their energy (calories or kilojoules) and protein requirements may be much higher than that of an active younger person just to prevent further muscle breakdown and weight loss. Disability and malnutrition are strongly related. Immobility with chronic illness in the elderly is associated with "hyper-catabolism" with an increased metabolic rate. The body uses up excessive amounts of protein from muscle to make energy, in combination with inadequate intake and the presence of inflammatory conditions or infections causing further muscle breakdown. These are the very types of patients who need almost double the amount of calories/kilojoules and protein than a younger fit person would require.

They consume much more energy and nutrients just to maintain balance and allow healing to take place. These frail elderly consume much more energy just to walk the same distance, and do the same daily activities as a younger fit person. They need to consume as much food as the young super fit Wests Tigers front row forward Rugby League players, which is 3 large hot meals a day plus lots of extra snacks just to maintain weight. Unfortunately many older people consume only a tiny breakfast, one slice of bread for lunch and a tea cup size dinner in the evening. This is self- starvation and will result in the downhill spiral of worsening health, muscle weakness, confusion, falls, ankle swelling, paper thin skin, leg ulcers, dehydration, infections and a presentation to the hospital Emergency Department.

Chronic conditions that cause need for larger intakes of calories and protein include:
- Heart Failure
- Chronic lung disease (Emphysema)
- Chronic inflammatory arthritis
- Parkinson's disease
- Dementia
- Walking and balance disorders
- Fractured hip or pelvis
- Chronic infections
- Chronic leg ulcers

## MUM HAS ALWAYS BEEN A SMALL EATER

Many older people commonly proudly exclaim that they have always been a "small eater" and wear this statement as a "badge of honour". It's a bit like saying that they have been smoking for 60 years! So what are they trying to tell us, that smoking is okay?

NO! Undereating is a very great risk to the older person's health. Malnutrition from undereating is one of the commonest causes for falls, infections, confusion and acute public hospital Emergency Department presentations for the elderly. Undereating and starvation are extremely common in people over 65 years of age. Many older women have grown up with the concept through women's magazines and attitudes in society that being thin is good. Delusions about skinny body figure and weight loss even occur in older people. I commonly see older women who are extremely thin and malnourished who still say they are overweight and need to cut back on what they eat! Obsessions about being thin, losing weight and eating very small meals may be the first sign of dementia.

Malnutrition is also worsened by families who lack insight into the nutritional requirement for frail older people. Many families still believe it is okay not to eat much as you get older. In fact they think it is a normal part of ageing which is completely wrong! Frail older people with multiple chronic illnesses need to eat more than double what a young fit footballer would be eating. This is just to meet their energy requirements and prevent muscle breakdown.

You don't get enough calories or energy from protein which is about 25% of the diet. Eating too much cheese and meat simply makes them too full too soon. Rather, they need a lot more calories from cakes, biscuits, chocolates, sweets, ice cream and desserts to stop the body breaking down muscle to make glucose for the brain and other key organs.

## UNDEREATING IS A MENTAL ILLNESS IN THE ELDERLY

Yes, this is definitely not normal behaviour. This usually occurs in frail older people with other illnesses or dementia. They may not be depressed. This food refusal, eating way less than they need to maintain health, and self- starvation is very common and leads to catastrophic outcomes such as-

- falls,
- worsening mobility,
- difficulty getting out of chairs,

- confusion (delirium),
- dehydration,
- infections,
- skin tears,
- pressure ulcers,
- Public Hospital Emergency Department presentations,
- Early Nursing Home admission.

The common unrealistic and ridiculous reasons why these elderly people refuse to eat when they are already starving themselves to death and rapidly losing weight include-

- I'm not hungry.
- I can't eat larger meals.
- I just don't want to eat.
- I don't need to eat much.
- I've always been a small eater.
- I don't need a lot of food.
- I don't do much so I don't need to eat.
- A small bikkie and a cup of tea is plenty for dinner.
- My main meal is dry crackers and a slice of cheese for lunch.
- I split my frozen meal in half- that's plenty.

There is usually no reason why non-demented older people cannot eat proper meals and have enough food! They just think it and believe it!

## MUM HAS HER MAIN MEAL AT 6PM

This is "red flag" warning sign that the older person is undereating and is malnourished. Older people commonly exclaim with pride that their "main meal" is in the evening, and a small meal anyway. These elderly tend to have very little for breakfast, no snacks during the day, only 1 slice of bread for a sandwich for lunch or a small cup of soup. Their dinner may be only a small serve of soup, a slice of bread and that's it. Many older people tend to collect and hoard their delivered meals in the fridge, dividing the already very small meal anyway into halves! They commonly divide a takeaway quarter BBQ chicken into 3 days of meals instead of eating the whole thing straight away. Or they just collect frozen meals in the freezer and never eat them! This can be the first sign of dementia. They should be having at least 3 hot meals a day and snacks in between to prevent weight loss, muscle breakdown and malnutrition. Hoarding uneaten meals in the fridge that go off may be the first sign of dementia.

## MY MOTHER EATS "HEALTHY FOODS"

Many of the frail older people that I see who exclaim proudly that they eat healthy foods are much more likely to end up in hospital as a result. Healthy foods such as salads, lean meats, low fat milk, dry biscuits and small serves do not give the frail older person enough calories and energy that they require. These so-called "healthy foods" simply accelerate the process of malnutrition, confusion, muscle weakness, falls and the risk for the public hospital Emergency Department presentation.

The best food for frail underweight malnourished older people are Polish Pierogi potato dumplings. They can be boiled and served with lashings of sour cream or fried in lots of butter and served with sour cream. They have lots of calories (kilojoules) for energy, are easy to swallow and eat, and taste fantastic! It is very much comfort food and provides better energy and food value than salads.

182

## I DON'T WANT TO COOK ANYMORE

This is a major warning sign of impending malnutrition and subsequent serious complications of undereating. When older people stop cooking and say that they are not hungry or just not interested in food, then this ends up becoming a crisis and an emergency. Why are they just not interested in good food and enjoy eating? The common answers are-

- Depression.
- Dementia.
- Chronic underlying untreated medical conditions.
- Chronic pain.
- Constipation.
- Chronic nausea.
- Dry mouth.
- Swallowing difficulties.
- Gastro-oesophageal reflux.
- Poor mobility.
- Social isolation.
- Adverse drug reactions.

These older people rapidly lose muscle strength and end up having difficulty getting out of a chair or just start falling. They can develop ankle swelling from severe malnutrition and skin bruising (brown staining) on their legs (shins) from loss of body fat and paper thin skin. If they continue to undereat and starve themselves, then they end up crossing the "Thin Red Line" and end up in the public hospital Emergency Department with falls, delirium, dehydration, infections and very high risk of ending up in a Nursing Home, losing their independence which are all completely preventable with better nutrition and simply eating better!

## MALNUTRITION IN DEMENTIA

One of the first signs of dementia is food refusal, eating smaller and smaller meals, and just loss of interest in food.

Dementia is the most common reason for elderly patients living in nursing homes to be spoon fed. This is usually a late complication in the course of dementia.

It is well recognised that weight loss in some dementia patients exceeds that predicted from inadequate dietary intake. This is because some dementia patients become "hypercatabolic", so burn up energy rapidly even when sedentary, and just continue to lose weight, even though they are eating adequate amounts of food.

Acute admission to hospital is a major risk factor for weight loss in frail and dementia patients.

There are other issues for malnutrition in dementia including:

- Forgetting to eat due to poor memory.
- Loss of smell and taste sensation.
- Difficulty recognising familiar foods.
- Dyspraxia or incoordination with eating.
- Holding utensils and cutting up food.
- Chewing and swallowing.
- Food refusal.
- Having very small meals.
- Poor dental and oral hygiene.
- Restlessness, unable to sit at dining table.

Offering finger food, regular snacks and small frequent serves of food may improve intake for people with advanced dementia. Writing down their favourite 10 savoury and sweet foods may help if they have to go to hospital or nursing home respite so that staff know what they actually like to eat.

Major risk factors for malnutrition in the elderly are social isolation, living alone, being housebound, poverty, difficulty shopping, chronic pain and excess alcohol intake.

We must always have a very high index of suspicion for malnutrition in our older patients, particularly those who end up in the acute hospital setting and those in nursing homes. Nutritional assessment is multi-factorial and management requires a multi-disciplinary approach, often with home assessments and in collaboration with the Dietitian, Physiotherapist and Speech Pathologist.

It is crucial that the underlying acute on chronic medical problems are accurately diagnosed, sorted out and properly treated. Poor dietary intake alone must not be blamed for the malnutrition.

## NUTRITION SCREENING TOOL

Simple screening tools can be very effective in identifying high risk patients. Some of the simple questions asked include:

- I have an illness or condition that may change the kind or amount of food I eat.
- I eat at least 3 meals per day.
- I eat fruit or vegetables most days.
- I eat dairy products most days.
- I have 3 or more glasses of alcohol.
- I have up to 8 cups of fluid per day including water, juice, tea or coffee.

- I have teeth, mouth or swallowing problems that make it harder for me to eat.
- I always have enough money to buy food.
- I eat alone most of the time.
- I take 3 or more different prescribed medications.
- Without wanting to, I have lost weight in the last 6 months.
- I am always able to shop, cook and feed myself.

This check list can alert families, Doctors and nurses to potential malnutrition problems. Nutritional screening should be a routine part of all medical assessments of the elderly.

Severely malnourished elderly people have a much higher risk of dying from their chronic medical problems than well-nourished older people. There are many reversible causes for a decreased appetite including too many medications, problems with teeth, mouth and swallowing, loss of taste, living alone, being housebound and chronic pain.

# THE IMPAIRED OLDER DRIVER

This topic generates much controversy among Doctors. Unfortunately many Doctors are reluctant to deal with the issue, so the common way of dealing with it is actually to ignore it.

There is no doubt that older people can still drive cars safely, even into their 90s. However, crash statistics show generally that drivers aged 85 or older have amongst the highest per kilometre crash rates and driving fatality rates. They suffer more severe injuries at lower crash velocities and with minor crashes. They are generally over-represented in traffic accident statistics and the fatality rate for older drivers is about 17 times higher than the rate for 25-65 year old age groups. Drivers 65 years and older make up about 15% of the population but are involved in about 20% of fatal crashes and 17% of pedestrian fatalities.

Death rates in drivers 65 years of age and older have increased by 10% in the last 10 years. The death rate for crashes in the 75 years and older group is much higher than both the middle age groups and the total. Figures in Australia are similar to other OECD countries.

Road crash injuries have a much worse impact on older people. A person aged 75 or older injured in a car crash usually has a much more severe injury and spends twice as long in hospital on average than younger drivers.

The number of older drivers on the road has increased, particularly for those 65 years and older by nearly 50% in the last decade. This reflects the ageing population in Australia and elsewhere. Old people are simply living longer and driving longer! About 20% of 70 year olds have some form of cognitive impairment. About 10% of older people develop mild cognitive impairment annually. The number of older drivers with mild cognitive impairment and unrecognised dementia is rapidly rising! I estimate that at least 10% of drivers over 70 years of age have unrecognised dementia and it may be even more than 25% for those drivers over 80 years.

The over 65 years population are growing faster than other age groups. Over 60% of people aged 75 years and over have a driving licence in Australia. I estimate that there are at least 160,000 drivers over 75 years of age on Australian roads with unrecognised dementia!

Even though older people tend to self-restrict their driving, they are still exposed to a higher number of crashes than younger drivers per kilometre driven. Older drivers are more commonly involved in crashes involving intersections and round-a-bouts. Older drivers in general, and especially male drivers are very reluctant to give up driving no matter how unwell or frail they are. They all say that they are good drivers!

In the last decade older drivers aged 60-74 years involved in serious crashes/injury have increased by 40%, and those aged 85 years or more have increased by 95%.

Frail older drivers are more likely to die in a car crash than younger drivers. Those drivers 85 years and older have more than 3 times the risk of dying in a car crash than for drivers aged less than 60 years.

Overall, drivers aged 75 years or more have a higher chance of being killed in a crash than any other age group for distance travelled. Most of these fatal crashes involve multiple vehicles, and occur at intersections or head on.

The major risk for crashes in the elderly are undiagnosed dementia and neurological conditions, those with multiple unmanaged co-morbidities and multiple adverse drug reactions. Together with hearing loss, loss of muscle strength and flexibility, slowed reflexes, these can cause slower reaction times, impaired visual perception and scanning, and impaired perceptions on the road.

Those people at risk of impaired driving include-
- Serious walking and balance disorders.
- Flexed posture, marked slowing of movement.
- Impaired righting reflexes.
- Restricted neck movements impeding lateral rotation to check for blind spots.
- Slowed information processing.
- Poor vision.
- Poor hearing.
- Vague and repetitive.
- Cognitive impairment.
- Poor memory.
- Poor attention.
- Poor insight.
- Poor judgement.
- Poor comprehension.
- Slowed reaction times.
- Poor coordination.
- Poor problem solving.
- Easily distracted.
- Muscle weakness.
- Taking multiple medications.

Patients with Alzheimer's dementia have a much higher crash risk than age-matched elderly controls. Statistics can be skewed because patients with dementia tend to restrict their driving and may be under-represented in studies.

Many studies of driving with cognitive impairment consistently demonstrate impaired performance in patients with dementia, compared to normal elderly drivers.

Driving is very much a cognitive or mental exercise.

Most elderly patients with Alzheimer's dementia lack insight into their cognitive impairments. They do not understand this. This is why self-assessment of driving doesn't work here! Similarly, many relatives also are unaware that driving is very much a cognitive or mental activity and they can't reconcile the fact that someone who is cognitively impaired or confused should not be allowed to drive a motor vehicle. There is very much the perception amongst families that they would like to see their elderly relative on the road for as long as possible, despite their cognitive impairment, risk of crashes and injury to themselves and others. Whilst they want to maintain their independence, they are simply putting the impaired older driver and the community at risk through increased crash risk from poor driving performance which has clearly been established in studies.

There is now quite strong evidence that the risk of motor vehicle accidents for drivers with dementia is significant, even in the early stages and gets worse as the disease progresses. Drivers with Alzheimer's dementia have nearly a 5 times crash risk compared to normal age match elderly controls.

This is not surprising, as even in early Alzheimer's dementia the patient would have had the neuropathology developing in their brain for at least 3 years prior to presentation to me. By the time they see me they usually have significant impairments in short-term memory, in other domains of the brain, and day-to-day living functions.

Safe driving cognitive performance requires-
- Fast speed of information processing.
- Quick reflexes.
- Accurate visual vigilance.
- Visuospatial orientation which is usually impaired in the early stages of dementia.
- Being able to maintain sustained attention and concentration without distraction.
- Simultaneous attention of more than 2 stimuli.
- Divided attention when needing to look to the left or to the right, behind or in front.
- Rapid change focus of concentration.
- Impaired judgement reduces the driver's ability to make appropriate decisions in complex traffic situations.
- Difficulty in coping with sudden changes or a new environment.
- Preserved short-term memory to remember speed limits and traffic signs.
- Judgement.

Overall you have to be super alert and very agile to drive a car safely, rather than being slothful, dithering, really slow in thinking and reflexes.

Drivers with dementia do not have the short-term memory to remember and process changes in traffic conditions, lights and signs.

There is still some controversy amongst Geriatricians and Neurologists, some of whom suggest it is okay for patients with Alzheimer's dementia to still drive motor vehicles. If that is the case, then when do they stop driving? Do you wait until they have an accident, kill someone on the road or injure themselves? I think the evidence is pretty clear now that this is a dangerous strategy.

## RESTRICTED DRIVERS LICENCE

The use of restricted or endorsed licences to restrict the distance travelled has not been proven to be a safe or effective strategy and commonly gives a false sense of security to drivers with dementia and their Doctors, based on the very erroneous expectation that people with dementia will not have problems if they remain in familiar surroundings. Almost all older drivers with restricted licences are medically unfit to drive! They are given these restricted licences as social excuse to prevent them being stranded without a car even though they are severely impaired and pose a major risk on the road.

Many of these older drivers with restricted licences have very poor vision and hearing, can barely walk with a frame, are extremely slow in mobility, reflexes and thinking, on multiple sedative medications and pain killers including narcotics, can barely turn their head to check blind spots, and are confused. The privilege to drive a car should not override the safe of the community. The increased crash risk for drivers with dementia remains, even though they may restrict their driving.

Also having somebody act like a "co-pilot" in the passenger seat to assist the driver with dementia is an unsafe practice and does not reduce the crash risk. Unfortunately I still see patients whose driving licence has been cancelled but they are still driving without a licence because of lack of insight, denial and memory loss. When they are challenged about this their common response is "I don't need a licence Doctor- I only drive locally down to the shops!"

## IDENTIFYING THE IMPAIRED OLDER DRIVER

Routine medical examinations frequently fail to diagnose or identify elderly drivers with dementia and poor driving habits, or those at higher crash risk. Increased crash risk is commonly associated with a lower mini mental state examination score, but this is not always the case.

When a spouse or family member tells me that the driving performance and behaviour is impaired, they are nearly always right. However, when they say that they are a good driver this is completely unreliable.

Of course the patients are generally very defensive and pro-active in stating that they are a good driver. I have never met an Australian older driver who says that his/her driving has become impaired. All Australian males say that they are good drivers! This is because the hallmark of Alzheimer's dementia is the lack of insight into their cognitive and functional impairments and decline.

Those elderly drivers who struggle to get in and out of their car, take forever to do so, have very poor balance and mobility, and use a walking frame are most likely to have significant neurological impairment affecting the speed of their reflexes, reaction times, information processing and safety with driving.

Cognitive screening should be routinely performed in all elderly drivers as part of their general medical assessments and screening for dementia.

I published a study on "Unrecognised Dementia in Older Drivers". Australasian Journal on Ageing 2003; 22; No.2: 106.(Ref 28). This was a retrospective audit of 598 geriatric medical hospital inpatients and home visit consultations were reviewed to see how many of these patients had the formal diagnosis of dementia but were still driving a motor vehicle. 56 (9% of patients) were identified out of the 598, with newly diagnosed dementia who were still driving a motor vehicle at the time of the Geriatric Medicine consultation. The average age was 80.4 years. Their average mini mental status score was only 20/30, with a score as low as 5/30 in one driver. They were all deemed to be not medically fit to drive a motor vehicle. Their driving had unfortunately not been addressed by the usual General Practitioner, despite being under regular review by the GP.

Of concern, the reasons for the Geriatric Medicine consultation were for memory loss, falls and balance disorders, delirium, agitation, paranoid delusions, benzodiazepine dependency, severe chronic lung disease, postural hypotension, dizziness and hallucinations.

This study illustrates how high a threshold and tolerance we have for chronic disability and impairment in older drivers.

Another one of my studies "Driving and Dementia: A Prospective Audit of Clients Referred to an Aged Care Assessment Team" - Australian Journal on Ageing V22: December 2003, 215-217. (Ref 27). Of 1203 people referred to an Aged Care Assessment Team,

100 (8% of these) were driving and 34% of those driving had some form of cognitive impairment, some of which was quite severe. The results of my study supported findings from other studies which suggested there was a small but significant number of elderly people with cognitive impairment who were still driving.

## WHY DON'T DOCTORS DEAL WITH IMPAIRED OLDER DRIVERS?

One may ask why are Doctors not dealing with the issue? In Australia it is not compulsory to deal with the impaired elderly driver (except in South Australia and the Northern Territory where mandatory reporting of impaired drivers is in place). Doctors are very reluctant to deal with the issue for fear of medical complaints against them if they confront an unsuspecting elderly patient about cancelling their driving licence, even though the Doctor is acting in the best interests of the patient and the community to maintain their safety. They are also fearful of damaging the Doctor-patient relationship. There is also enormous pressure from the patient and the relatives to keep older people driving on the road. In fact many Doctors still believe that it is safe to drive a car even with early Alzheimer's Dementia and do not recommend licence cancellation.

I studied this issue in a survey of General Practitioners' attitudes to older drivers on the NSW Central Coast. Australian Journal on Aging V21: 2: 2002 p 98-100. (Ref 24). I surveyed 275 GPs with regard to their attitudes to older drivers. Of concern, 61% of GPs allowed an older driver with mild Alzheimer's disease to still drive a motor vehicle. 21% of GPs would allow the frail medically unfit driver to still drive with a restricted licence locally if there was no public transport nearby. Only 41% of GPs thought they had enough training to make an appropriate medical driver assessment. Only 29% of GPs routinely ask about driving habits and medical fitness to drive in all of their older patients. Over 55% of GPs felt that there should be another medical body to oversee all medical driver assessments rather than the GP to protect them from damaging the Doctor/patient relationship and complaints.

## TYPICAL RESPONSES WHEN DRIVING LICENCES ARE CANCELLED

From one of my studies I summarised the typical responses from demented drivers when confronted about giving up their licence, and particularly with males, they always had the same response.

- I have a gold licence you know. (In NSW Australia this means they have just paid for a licence for 5 years.)

- I have been driving for 50 years you know! However, it doesn't matter how long the person has been driving, it only matters what the driver's medical fitness and their driving performance is now.

- I have never had an accident!

- I can't survive without my car!

- How could you do this to me?

- I will see my Solicitor/Lawyer about this.

- I am not going to give up my licence.

- I might as well jump off a cliff if I can't drive!

Fortunately most of the patients I deal with in cancelling their driving licence still come back to see me.

## I JUST PASSED MY DRIVING TEST

I frequently see patients with fairly advanced dementia and confusion who are still driving their motor vehicles and would you believe have just passed the State Government driving test! These impaired older drivers must not be allowed to drive for both their safety and the safety of the community. It is a real challenge for the Doctor to convince these confused older drivers that they are no longer able to drive their motor vehicle despite passing this State Government driving test. These driving tests do not identify cognitive impairment in the older driver. The patient's lack of insight due to their dementia means that they frequently ignore the medical recommendation and go on to drive, even when their licence has been cancelled.

Common responses include:

- I just passed my driving test.
- I only drive to the shops.
- I don't need a licence to drive short distances.

## THE RAMP TEST

I have a gentle sloping ramp in front of my Private Consulting Rooms to the front door. When I see older people struggling to walk along it, particularly those with walking frames who are very slow and unsteady, this indicates that they should not be driving a car! Severe mobility impairments are commonly associated with underlying neurodegenerative (brain) disorders with poor balance, very slowed reflexes, cognitive impairments and dementia. These older people have severely impaired coordination, speed of thinking and reaction times. These neurological functions are essential for safe driving. These impaired older people are unsafe to drive a car!

## MY MOTHER NEEDS HER CAR

I frequently see elderly people who were referred to me because they are confused and unable to manage alone at home. Then when I diagnose them with significant dementia and confusion and tell them that they are no longer medically fit to drive a motor vehicle, their daughter usually says to me "You can't do that!" "My Mother needs her car".

You've got to be kidding me! Many families think it is OK for a confused older person to drive a car! Work that out! They can't look after themselves alone at home, they can't even use a microwave oven yet their family still think it is okay for them to drive a motor vehicle! The lack of insight from patient and family is extremely worrying. These impaired older drivers can barely walk, are so slow in thinking, movement and reflexes, vague and confused, yet family who insist that they can still drive a car commonly say "Mum is pretty good for her age, very sharp mentally!" indicating severe denial of their physical and cognitive impairments. This indicates a gross lack of respect for the safety of other drivers and pedestrians! They don't even know the speed limits outside schools in school zone times and in built-up areas!

When I first started private practice, families would thank me enormously when I cancelled the licence of impaired confused older drivers, but of late I see the complete opposite in that families insist that their frail, unwell and confused relatives still drive their car when it is unsafe to do so. Most people do not understand the high crash risk and danger that these impaired older drivers pose when still driving. There seems to be a very high tolerance for drivers with severe impairments in Australia and a lack of respect for the complexities and risks of driving a car.

This is an ongoing huge issue for the patients, GPs and their families. The patients and families can't reconcile why they can't drive when they have just passed their routine State Government driving test at the age of 85.

## STATE GOVERNMENTS FAILED OLDER DRIVER ASSESSMENTS

Unfortunately the State Government Driving Licence test is a failed system and doesn't have a low enough threshold to detect impaired cognition and dementia in these drivers. It is a simple steering test of a car in a quiet traffic situation. The patient with dementia can still drive and steer the car adequately in a short period of time. This is because the older driver aged 85 and older usually has been driving for over 60 years and has very much a "structural and procedural memory" embedded in their brain so that driving becomes almost "automatic", but without the awareness or the visual vigilance and other cognitive functions necessary for safe driving to reduce their crash risk. So many people with early Alzheimer's dementia and those with even more significant cognitive impairment can still pass the State Government driving test!

Given their lack of insight, this is why self-assessment does not work for the elderly and they do not readily give up their driving licence for fear of being stranded or socially isolated.

The bottom line is that State Governments should not be dishing out these driving licences to impaired older drivers. I recommend that all drivers aged 70 and over should have an annual memory test. If they don't get 100% they should be referred to a Geriatrician for further cognitive assessment before they can get their driving licence.

This topic generally generates headlines. Back in 1997 I estimated there were at least 80,000 drivers with dementia on the NSW State roads in Australia.

I routinely see elderly drivers over 85 years of age who have very significant dementia, but have retained excellent language and social skills to hide their significant dementia, so that they do present superficially "well'. These people are so impaired that they are unable to draw numbers on a clock face, are disorientated in time and cannot tell me their home address, yet are still driving a motor vehicle!

The clock drawing test, although it is non-specific, is a very good screening test for cognitive impairment and correlates well with dementia. It is a paradox that these patients who are unable to draw numbers on a clock face are allowed to drive a car in complex traffic situations, putting themselves and the public at risk. It is clear that dementia in older drivers is a common problem. The dementia is not screened for, it is underdiagnosed and undertreated. The current licensing situation in Australia is totally inadequate to deal with the rapidly ageing population and the disabilities associated with multiple chronic medical problems and dementia in the older population.

State Government Licensing Authorities who hand out driving licences to older drivers must take responsibility and deal with the problem, and develop cognitive screening procedures before giving out these licences. They should not be delegating driving assessments to Doctors who are not only reluctant to deal with this complex issue, have no training in medical driver assessments, but also may have a conflict of interest in keeping their patients happy and maintaining a positive Doctor-patient relationship.

It should not be up to the Doctor to sort this out, or to be held responsible or to wait for the crisis to occur.

## EXCUSES TO KEEP IMPAIRED OLDER DRIVERS ON THE ROAD

Many families try to keep their elderly parents and relatives driving just to please them and avoid an unpleasant argument. Get a load of what some families say about their older relatives who are confused, impaired physically and mentally but are still driving- these are typical classic responses:
-he only drives slowly.
-he doesn't need to know the speed limits because he only drives to the shops.
-I take over the driving when he gets too confused.
-I tell him where to go, when to turn and what to do.
-I help her get into and out of the car.

-she only drives when the roads are quiet without much traffic.
-she gets dizzy and is very unsteady when walking but no problems driving the car.
-what's memory got to do with driving?
-you can't stop him driving- he needs the car!
-he is a good driver!
-I haven't noticed any memory loss or confusion.
-she needs help to manage alone at home but she can still drive her car!
-he has been driving all his life and never had an accident.
-she is OK just driving locally down to the shops.
-he always drinks at least 1 bottle of wine every night but it never affects his driving.
-he lives for driving, it will ruin him if he can't drive.
-why can't he drive just because he is confused and forgetful?
-her morphine and sleeping pills never affect her driving, just makes her sleepy during the day.

## **I ONLY DRIVE TO THE SHOPS LOCALLY**

Many impaired older drivers and their families insist they should still be allowed to drive because they only drive a few kilometres to the local shops. This is even so when they have significant confusion and memory loss. Driving a motor vehicle requires a person to be cognitively intact and not confused. The distance travelled is irrelevant and only driving short distances when you are impaired and confused does not mean that it is a safe practice. The risk to the driver and the community is just as significant wherever they drive. Many car accidents involving elderly drivers occur only a few kilometres from their home.

Most patients and families under-recognise the significant neurological/brain skills required to drive a motor vehicle. Driving is very much a cognitive exercise and not a physical exercise. Because the older person is physically fit but very confused, families think that is still okay for them to drive a motor vehicle when it is not!

## MISTAKING ACCELERATOR PEDAL FOR BRAKE PEDAL

If an older driver reverses at high speed and crashes into a shop front or fence because they pressed the accelerator pedal instead of the brake pedal, then this definitely means they should not be driving! It is not possible to mistake the pedals in a car unless you are impaired in some way. The brain and nerves in your legs are so in tune as to what you feel with your feet and where they are positioned that you can't get this wrong. Even when you are sitting at a meeting with others and your foot brushes against another person under the table you immediately react, move your foot away and say excuse me. Those impaired older drivers with dementia, on multiple sedative drugs, slowed reflexes and impaired peripheral nerve sensation in the feet should not be driving. This is one big mistake, a warning sign where one strike and you are out- no more driving!

## TAKE THE CAR KEYS OFF MOTHER

Many families do not want to upset their elderly mother or father who are still driving, when clearly not medically fit to drive. Rather than confront them they just ignore the problem and let them drive. However, to be fair to families, I have seen several cases where the daughter has removed the keys and the car from their mother's access. Their mother has then made a formal complaint to the Police and the daughter has been charged with car theft. This is despite the daughter or son acting in the best interests of the person and the community to protect everyone from injury from an impaired older driver.

There are many medically unfit older drivers who simply refuse to stop driving when told by their families to stop. This is because of lack of insight and self-awareness particularly with dementia. So when the Doctor doesn't cancel their licence, and they refuse to listen to the family and there is no Enduring Guardianship then they are heading for a crisis and a crash! So we are left with many such dangerous older drivers unaware of the grave risks that they pose to others and there is nothing the family can do.

Even if the impaired older driver still drives without a licence, all the Police will do is to pull them over and issue them an Infringement Notice if they are caught and then they will keep driving without a licence because the impaired older driver lacks insight into the issues and has no memory of the event. Even the dodgy older drivers who clearly pose a risk to other drivers and pedestrians will only be issued an Infringement Notice if they are crossing their lane, not giving way and will simply keep on driving. The system doesn't identify these high risk drivers and refer them for further appropriate medical assessments. Therefore, it is very difficult for families to intervene unless they have Enduring Guardianship to be able to make these difficult decisions.

## MEDICATIONS CAN IMPAIR DRIVING PERFORMANCE

Medications that can affect driving performance include cardiac medications which can lower blood pressure and cause dizziness, sedatives, sleeping pills, anti-depressants, psychotropics, narcotic analgesics and other pain killers, which can make the person drowsy, confused, all of which can impair reflexes, concentration, information processing and driving performance. Then there is a risk of drug interactions and adverse drug reactions when older drivers are on more than 4 prescribed medications.

## THE TRIGGERS FOR MEDICAL ASSESSMENTS OF OLDER DRIVERS

- Slowing of thinking.
- Poor short-term memory.
- Falls, faints, dizziness, low blood pressure.
- Slowing of walking and movements.
- Poor vision.
- Poor hearing.
- Recent confusion/ delirium.
- Taking multiple medications.
- Struggling at home alone.
- Reports from family or friends that driving behaviour is erratic and unsafe.
- Evidence of frequent "dents", "dings", "bumps", "scratches' or more serious damage to the car.
- Risky and dangerous driving behaviours such as speeding, near misses, not giving way, veering out of lane
- Getting easily agitated or aggressive.
- Getting lost on familiar routes.
- Reacting very slowly to dangerous traffic situations.

- Frequently forgetting where the car was parked.
- Driving with head below the steering wheel level so they can't really see properly around them.
- Taking forever to get into and out of the car.
- Mistaking the accelerator for the brake pedal.

It still must be emphasised that I am talking about the impaired older driver. The majority of older drivers (70%) do not have issues with their physical or mental health or driving.

## OCCUPATIONAL THERAPY DRIVING ASSESSMENT:

The Occupational Therapy driving assessment is still regarded as the "gold standard" when there are doubts about driving capacity and performance in the older patient. Unfortunately I don't think it has much role in the patient with dementia. Even those patients with dementia whom I have seen still pass the OT driving test which shows the test has a very high threshold (not very sensitive) for detecting any impairments.

Even somebody with significant dementia whom I would deem to be medically unfit to drive a motor vehicle can still drive, steer the car and pass the test.

Therefore, I only refer patients to the Occupational Therapy driving assessment who have mild cognitive impairment, but no formal diagnosis of dementia who are otherwise medically fit to drive a motor vehicle, but there are some concerns about their current physical or cognitive state. Unfortunately many Doctors use the Occupational Therapy driving assessment as a substitute decision making process because they are not prepared to make the decision about medical fitness to drive themselves, but rather devolve it to the Occupational Therapist.

# PERI-OPERATIVE MEDICAL ASSESSMENT

With the ageing of the population more older people now are undergoing general anaesthetics and major surgery. Evidence is accumulating that comprehensive holistic Geriatric Medical care and assessment before and after surgery makes a huge difference to the outcome of the surgery, avoids complications, reduces the risk of post-operative delirium and post-operative cognitive decline.

In my Geriatric Medical Practice I work very closely now with Orthopaedic Surgeons, Plastic Surgeons and General Surgeons to assist in the peri-operative medical care of elderly surgical patients.
So what is peri-operative care?

- pre-operative comprehensive medical assessment, focusing on management and appropriate optimising of treatment of the intercurrent chronic active medical problems.
- pre-operative cognitive assessment.
- screening for delirium.
- minimising post-operative delirium and post-operative cognitive decline.
- reviewing all their medications.
- assessing their nutrition to prevent post-operative malnutrition.
- early mobility post- op.
- safe and adequate pain management.
- to allow for the best surgical and medical outcome following the surgery.

The days when complex frail older patients can be operated on by a Surgeon alone, independently without being part of a multi-disciplinary medical team with the Geriatrician are rapidly fading. The multiple "Single Organ Doctor" consultations for post-operative complications such as the heart Doctor, the kidney Doctor, the blood Doctor, the lung Doctor and the nerve Doctor do not result in the best health outcome for the elderly surgical patient without involving a multi-disciplinary team, and someone taking control of their medical care, their overall treatment and outcomes. It is also much more cost effective (much much cheaper!) for hospitals and Government Health Departments to have a Geriatrician overseeing post-operative care rather than multiple single organ Doctors.

Surgeons must screen for cognitive impairment and post operative delirium risk before they operate on patients over 65 years. They must also closely review and monitor the patient in the immediate post operative period for delirium. Relegating this to Junior Medical Staff in hospital is just not good enough! All Surgeons who operate on older patients must have training in Geriatric Medicine and work closely with a Geriatrician in a multi-disciplinary care setting to achieve safe and effective surgical outcomes. One may argue, do we want surgeons to be very good at just operating? NO! They also must be very good at post-operative care and pre-operative assessments of patients to reduce post-operative complications.

There should be a clear overall plan before major surgery as to how to manage fluid balance, post-operative anaemia, blood transfusions, post-operative pain, drugs, early mobility and preventing adverse drug reactions, and post-operative cognitive decline.

There is no point in operating on elderly patients if the outcome is poor because of multiple complications such as post op delirium, falls, malnutrition, poor mobility and adverse drug reactions. It's a bit like saying "well the operation was a success, but what about the patient"?

Current evidence-based medicine tells us that Geriatrician-led peri-operative care reduces post-operative complications and mortality and results in a shorter length of hospital stay, less health care costs, and positive surgical and medical outcomes for the patient.

# CAPACITY TO CONSENT

Even with cognitive impairment and Alzheimer's dementia, some patients retain the capacity to consent to some issues. Consent is really task specific. The elderly person may not cope with complex legal documents or issues, but may be able to cope with simple decisions. Their capacity to consent would need to be assessed by the Geriatrician at the time, dealing with the matter at hand.

I always encourage families of older patients to get formal Enduring Guardianship and Enduring Power of Attorney as soon as possible whilst they are still able to do so. Once the patient has lost the capacity, this can cause huge complications for the family trying to assist the elderly patient who becomes confused, agitated, resistive to outside help, and who can no longer manage their finances, their daily life affairs or make appropriate decisions about their medical treatment and where they should be living.

To have the capacity to consent to Enduring Guardianship and Power of Attorney the person must be alert, not in delirium and should be orientated in time and place, aware of the issues that face them, the choices available to them and the consequences of their choices. In addition, with regard to Enduring Power of Attorney which is a legal construct anyway, the person needs to be aware that these documents are-
- only effective whilst the person is alive and has no effect after their death.
- they can revoke the Power of Attorney at any stage, as long as they have the mental capacity.
- the Power of Attorney is giving another person authority and that will extend after the person has

lost mental capacity to invoke the Enduring document.
- Enduring Power of Attorney is giving power to another person to manage the elderly person's financial affairs.
- to make decisions about buying and selling property.
- disposing and withdrawal of money, buying and selling shares, acting in their best interests.

With regard to Enduring Guardianship-
- it is giving authority to another person to make decisions about their life affairs.
- their place of living.
- their medical treatment when they no longer have the capacity to do so.

To be capable of granting Enduring Power of Attorney or Enduring Guardianship, the elderly person must understand the nature and effect of the document when explained to them. The person must be able to take in what was being explained to them and be able to demonstrate their understanding by communicating this back to the explainer.

In terms of a Will, whether or not the elderly person has the relevant mental capacity to be able to make a Will is dependent on-
- their ability to understand what a Will is,
- their ability to understand the extent of the property which he or she is disposing of by a Will,
- to be able to comprehend and appreciate the claims to which he or she ought to give effect to
- that there is no disorder of thinking that will prejudice their affections, pervert their sense of right or prevent the exercise of their natural faculties,

- and in particular that there is no delusion influencing them in disposing of their property and bringing about disposal of it, which if they had the capacity would not have been made.

Unfortunately, all too often I see elderly patients coming to see me when it is too late for them to make or change a Will, or to make up a new Enduring Guardianship or Power of Attorney. Then both the patient and family end up in a crisis during acute illness when nobody can make sensible decisions about the elderly patient's finances, medical treatment for place of living.

The alternative then is for the family to apply to the Guardianship Tribunal/the Court to become the legal Guardian.

## LOSS OF INSIGHT

The loss of insight into an older person's care needs is the most challenging and life-threatening situation an older person may have. Loss of insight is one of the hallmarks of early Alzheimer's dementia. The person loses their capacity to make rational decisions about their life affairs, place of living or medical treatment. They are therefore unable to understand when they require more help or a medical assessment. They make the wrong food choices and undereat, resulting in malnutrition and falls. They refuse to stop driving, as they have lost the capacity to understand that they pose a risk to themselves and others due to their frailty and cognitive impairment. They refuse outside support services when they clearly need extra help to stay independent at home. They refuse to go into Residential Aged Care when clearly they can no longer manage at home.

Without a pre-existing Enduring Guardianship or Power of Attorney, then the choices that families can make are extremely limited. If their elderly mother or father become aggressive or resistive to any help or interventions, then all the family can do is to wait for the crisis and until they cross the "Thin Red Line" when they end up in the public hospital Emergency Department in crisis. If they had the Enduring Guardianship and Power of Attorney organised earlier, then the family could make appropriate decisions to assist their frail, unwell, elderly parents before they end up in a crisis situation.

# ANAEMIA

Anaemia means that the "red blood cell count", or the level of the protein haemoglobin in red cells which carries oxygen through the body, is lower than normal which commonly results in adverse symptoms in the elderly.

Anaemia is not normal in the elderly, but is a common problem. It usually indicates that the person is unwell and may reflect serious underlying diseases. In those aged 85 and older the prevalence of anaemia exceeds 20% and in those elderly in Residential Aged Care settings such as hostels and nursing homes, the prevalence of anaemia can be above 60%. Anaemia is commonly ignored, underdiagnosed and undertreated in the elderly!

Numerous studies have shown that anaemia is an independent predictor of bad health outcomes in the elderly. The mortality risk is significantly higher in older anaemic adults, they die sooner.

Anaemia in the elderly is associated with significant functional impairments in day-to-day living including-

- Worsening breathlessness on minimal effort.
- Chest pain.
- Worsening heart failure.
- Worsening kidney failure.
- Dizziness.
- Falls.
- Confusion.
- Depression.
- General functional decline.
- Reduced exercise tolerance/distance walked.

- Increased risk for hospital Emergency Department presentation.
- Longer length of hospital stay.
- Increased mortality (death rate is doubled).

It can contribute to delirium and worsen dementia. Pre-operative anaemia before the elderly have major surgery is also associated with an increased complication rate after surgery including increased rates of post-operative infections.

Even mild anaemia is common with haemoglobin less than the normal 13g/dl for males and less than 12g/dl for females. This can cause significant problems for the elderly.

Anaemia should never be regarded as a normal part of ageing. It is always caused by underlying illness and may be multi-factorial in nature. A common cause of anaemia that I see includes iron deficiency anaemia which usually means bleeding from the gastrointestinal tract either from the bowel, the oesophagus, stomach or duodenum. The causes of such bleeding include Aspirin use, NSAIDs (arthritis pills), anti-coagulants, peptic ulcers, reflux oesophagitis, gastric cancer, bowel cancer, bowel polyps and haemorrhoids. Anaemia maybe the first sign of underlying bowel cancer. Where possible the patient should have an accurate diagnosis with endoscopy or colonoscopy rather than just an iron infusion or blood transfusion without determining the underlying cause of the anaemia, otherwise it is likely to recur and if underlying cancer then the outcome will be bad.

Iron deficiency even without anaemia may also be the first sign of bowel cancer in the elderly. Iron deficiency with or without anaemia makes heart failure worse. Severe iron deficiency can be treated with an intravenous iron infusion. Oral iron tablets can be very constipating in the elderly. Iron deficiency should not be blamed on poor diet in the elderly. It is commonly caused by other serious underlying medical problems.

The most common type of anaemia in the elderly is "anaemia of chronic disease" which caused by multiple underlying chronic medical conditions including:

- Chronic kidney disease.
- Malnutrition.
- Chronic infections.
- Myelodysplasia-impaired bone marrow function, inability to produce red blood cells.
- Malignancy affecting the bone marrow-myeloma or leukaemia.

Doctors commonly allow older patients to have severe anaemia (a very low Hb or haemoglobin) without giving them a blood transfusion. Hb lower than 10g/L commonly causes severe symptoms in the frail elderly. They are poorly tolerant of severe anaemia and should be transfused early.

Anaemia should be actively investigated, diagnosed and managed, as older people can suffer significant symptoms and impairment of day-to-day function with even mild anaemia. They can have dramatic symptomatic, functional improvement and much better quality of life with active treatment of anaemia. It should not be ignored in the elderly!

# THE FUTURE OF MEDICINE

My vision for the future of Medicine for all people 70 years of age and over includes:

- Comprehensive Geriatric Medicine Assessment.
- Cognitive assessments to screen for delirium and dementia.
- Lying and standing BP measurements.
- Weight documented and calculated renal (kidney) function for age and weight for safe drug prescribing.
- Review of all medications, side effects and potential drug to drug interactions.
- Nutritional screening and Body Mass Index.
- Prioritising nutritional services and Dieticians at the top of the tree as the most important services in every hospital and nursing home.
- Assessment of balance and falls risk.
- Assessment of medical fitness to drive a car.
- Focus on holistic comprehensive general medicine, not the single organ approach.
- Assessing the whole patient, not just a single organ, and how multiple medical problems are affecting the general function and quality of life of the patient.
- Getting rid of single organ Doctors and single organ medicine- every Doctor to practise comprehensive holistic general medicine.
- All Doctors to provide home visit service for those elderly who can't get to rooms.
- All Surgeons operating on people over 70 years to work with a Geriatrician and provide comprehensive peri-operative care dealing

with all of the patient's medical issues, not just doing an operation.

- All Surgeons operating on people over 70 years to spend at least 12 months working with a Geriatrician for formal training in Geriatric Medicine.
- Hospitals and State Health Departments run by a committee of General Physician (Geriatrician), General Surgeon and Nurse reporting to the State Premier or State Governor, not run by administrators, bureaucrats, health economists or Health Ministers who have no medical qualifications.
- Health system to recognise the complexity of Geriatric Medicine, reward and provide incentives for comprehensive holistic general medical care, spending time with patients, rather than seeing multiple patients every few minutes just looking at one thing only.
- All Nursing Homes attached to Public Hospitals to provide comprehensive medical services to nursing home patients. Why should these patients miss out on good medical care just because they are in a nursing home?
- Doctors to involve family when appropriate taking into account patient wishes, consent and privacy laws.
- All drivers 70 years and over to have annual cognitive screen/memory test, and if impaired then Geriatrician review for safety of driving.
- Encourage all patients to have Enduring Guardianship and Enduring Power of Attorney.
- Encourage all patients to have an Advanced Care Plan-end of life decision making document.

# WHAT IS MULTIDISCIPLINARY HOLISTIC CARE?

## THE GERIATRICIAN

- A Physician who specialises in the medical care of the elderly. The Geriatrician provides holistic general medical care for the elderly, focuses on improving the symptoms and general function of frail complex elderly patients with multiple Geriatric syndromes such as
  - Confusion
  - Falls
  - Walking and balance disorders
  - Malnutrition
  - Swallowing disorders
  - Multiple medications and adverse drug reactions
  - Incontinence
  - Chronic pain

- They focus on managing acute on chronic medical conditions in elderly patients and improving physical, psycho-social and functional outcomes with appropriate treatment. Geriatricians look at the "whole patient", not a specific organ and deal with how the patient's diseases relate to their day-to-day function and difficulties managing at home.

- Geriatricians like to involve family where privacy laws permit and usually work closely with a multi-disciplinary team which involves:

- Specialist Geriatrics Practice Nurse, Physiotherapist, Occupational Therapist, Speech Pathologist, Dietitian.

- The Geriatrician works closely with General Practitioners (Primary Care Physicians) and other referring medical and surgical Specialists.

- Provides peri-operative care for general surgical and orthopaedic patients.

- Communication with GPs on discharge to handover ongoing medical care plans.

- Provides comprehensive Medical Discharge Summary faxed / emailed to the GP and other key health care workers involved in patient's ongoing care to maintain the good health outcomes.

## SPECIALIST GERIATRICS PRACTICE NURSE:

- Assists Geriatrician in coordination of medical care of the elderly inpatients.

- Assists in obtaining collateral history from relatives and friends regarding pre-existing physical and cognitive function when needed.

- Collating past medical history from multiple sources including other Specialists and previous Hospital admissions.

- Assists with cognitive screening and assessments.

- Assists in organising investigations.

- Updates families on patient's progress.

- Co-ordinates comprehensive discharge arrangements, care packages and follow-up appointments.

- Assists families to arrange respite care at home or in Residential Aged Care.

- Organises permanent Residential Aged Care (hostels and nursing homes).

## PHYSIOTHERAPIST:

- Multicomponent exercise programmes consisting of balance, resistance, walking, and gait retraining for the frail elderly, focusing on improving balance and maximising mobility, endurance, and functional independence.

- Improving and maintaining transfers from sit to stand from bed, chair and toilet, mobility, balance, exercise tolerance, strength of upper and lower limbs, particularly quadriceps strength, reducing falls risk and improving safety in the home environment.

- Measuring patients for Hip Protector underwear to reduce the risk of hip fracture with falls.

- Assessments for walking aids.

- Home based Physio assessments and treatments have been shown to reduce falls risks in the frail elderly.

## OCCUPATIONAL THERAPIST:

- Comprehensive assessments of frail aged patients, to maximise independence in activities of daily living.

- Specialises in activities of daily living such as dressing and showering, improving instrumental activities of daily living such as managing the household generally, including meal preparation and household appliances.

- Home visits to reduce falls risk and assess the home environment for home modifications such as installation of ramps, rails, remodelling of bathrooms to allow better entry in people who have balance problems and assessing the falls risk at home, shower hoses, chairs to improve independence.

- Providing equipment for those who are disabled such as adjusted cutlery for people with deforming arthritis in their upper limbs, cups with lids if they have a tremor causing spilling, gadgets, jar openers and improving fine hand function.

- Post-surgical assessment of general function and mobility. Focus on safe transfers out of bed, managing personal care whilst in hospital, falls risk assessment and equipment needed at home to stay independent.

Home visits by Occupational Therapists have also been shown to reduce the falls risk in elderly patients.

## SPEECH PATHOLOGIST:

- Assesses and manages swallowing problems in the elderly to reduce the risk of silent aspiration (food and fluid going down the wrong way into the lungs) and its complications (chest infections, pneumonia).

- Recommends the most appropriate consistency of food and fluid for safe swallowing. This may mean at times thickened fluids and finely cut-up meals with gravy or puree meals when needed to improve swallowing and reduce choking and silent aspiration.

- Works closely with Dietician to maximise nutrition, hydration and safe swallowing.

- Recommends the safest way of swallowing pills for patients with swallowing disorders. Sometimes this means taking pills with custard or yoghurt to reduce choking.

- Supervises modified Barium Video swallow Xrays to accurately diagnose and treat swallowing impairments and silent aspiration, and to be able to advise on the correct posture and head position when eating and drinking, best food and fluid consistency to ensure safe swallowing.

- Manages speech and communication disorders in the elderly.

# DIETITIAN:

- Specialist care of frail elderly with malnutrition.

- Nutritional screening and assessments of the elderly using validated assessment tools.

- Pre-operative nutritional screening to identify those at risk of malnutrition in the post-operative period.

- Appropriate dietary interventions including high protein, high energy diets and supplements.

- Management of Diabetic diets.

- Management of complex diets in heart failure with salt restrictions, kidney stones, potassium and calcium restrictions when needed.

- Works closely with the Speech Pathologist to improve nutritional state and dietary intake of the frail elderly who have swallowing difficulties.

# Dr PETER LIPSKI's AWARDS

- Director of Clinical Training Award for the Outstanding Clinical Teacher of the year Concord Hospital Sydney 1991.

- Doctor's Doctor Award teacher most valued by Junior Medical Staff, Central Coast Area Health Service NSW 1997 and 1999.

- The Post Graduate Medical Council of New South Wales Award in recognition of an outstanding commitment to Junior Doctor's post graduate education, training and supervision 1999.

- Highly Commended Award for Doctor's Doctor most valued by Junior Medical staff, Central Coast Health NSW 2001.

- Highly Commended Award for Doctor's Doctor most valued by Junior Medical staff, Central Coast Health NSW 2002.

# Dr PETER LIPSKI's MEDIA PRESENTATIONS and PUBLICATIONS

## MEDIA

"Nutrition checks for Elderly". Central Coast Express Advocate 15 Nov, 1995.

"Warning 80,000 Drivers with Dementia on the Roads". Sydney Morning Herald, August 22, 1997.

"Road R-Age". Central Coast Express Advocate 29 Aug, 1997.

"GPs in Dementia Dilemma". Central Coast Express. 5 July, 2002.

"Older drivers". 730 Report. ABC TV 2002.

Channel 9 Today Show TV interview- Drivers with Dementia 2005.

"Fed or Dead": Many older Australians are malnourished, and experts suspect some may even be starving to death: The Weekend Australian April 22-23, 2006.

"The Elderly Starved of Nutrition in Homes". - The Weekend Australian April 22-23, 2006.

"Stop Signs- When older drivers become a danger". Weekend Herald Newcastle Saturday, 9 June, 2007.

"Nutrition for older people". ABC Radio Central West. 11 July 2008.

"Frail elderly given new lease on life at holistic unit". Central Coast Express Advocate. 21 Oct 2008.

"New Age Longevity". Central Coast Express. 14 Nov, 2012.

"Adverse Drug Reaction Danger to the Elderly". Central Coast Express. 15 March, 2013.

ABC Central Coast Radio interview 26 March 2019.

Book dispels myths about health issues due to "old age". Australian Ageing Agenda. 24 April, 2019.

"Old age will not kill you. Western Medicine is mistreating older people. Dr Peter Lipski is fed up with the way our health care system is treating older Australians and has lifted the lid on misdiagnosis, malnutrition and other harmful medical myths." Daily Telegraph. 10 June 2019.

"You are never too old to be treated", says Geriatrician. Bad Medicine. Central Coast Express. 13 June, 2019.

Book review. Chicklitcafe.com 26 Jan 2020.

It's never too late to treat an older person. On The Coast Over 55. Issue 42, July/August 2021. P18-19.

## PRESENTATIONS

1. Lipski PS, Kelly PJ, James OFW. "Prevalence of Bacterial Contamination in the Small Bowel in the Elderly. Is it necessarily pathological?" (Oral & poster presentation, World Congress of Gastroenterology, Sydney, 27-28 August 1990.) PROC - World Congresses, Gastroenterology 1990; pp 536.

2. Lipski PS, Thomas JE, Eastman EJ, Kelly PJ, James OFW. "Association of Helicobacter Pylori in Bacterial

Contamination of the Small Bowel". (Poster presentation, World Congress of Gastroenterology, Sydney, 30 August 1990.) PROC - World Congresses, Gastroenterology 1990; pp 1948.

3. Lipski PS, Kelly PJ, James OFW. "Is Bacterial Contamination of the Small Bowel Common in the Elderly? If so, is it important?" (Oral presentation, British Geriatric Society Annual Autumn Scientific Meeting, Kensington Town Hall, London, 19 October 1990.) Age and Ageing 1991; 20: SUPPL 1:P6.

4. Lipski PS, Torrance A, Kelly PJ, James OFW. "Dietary Intake in Nutritional State of Fit Community Elderly versus Elderly Long Stay Hospital Patients versus Young Fit Subjects". (Oral presentation, Australian Association of Gerontology, Annual National Conference, Sheraton Wentworth Hotel, Sydney, 24 October 1991.) PROC - Aust. Ass. Gerontol. 1991.

5. Lipski PS. "The Consequences of Undernutrition in the Elderly". (Oral presentation, The Nutrition Society of Australia, 19th Annual Scientific Meeting, Melbourne, 27 September 1995.) PROC - Nutrition Society of Australia. Vol. 19: pp 146-151.

6. Lipski PS. "Recent Advances in Undernutrition in the Elderly". (Platform presentation for The Australian Society for Geriatric Medicine, Annual Scientific Meeting, Adelaide 1997.)

7. Lipski PS, Irvine W. "Dementia Drivers - A Cause for Concern". Abstract 875. (Platform presentation for the 16th Congress of International Association of Gerontology 1997, Adelaide, South Australia.)

8. Lipski PS. "Impaired Older Driver". Presented to Joint Standing Committee on Road Safety, NSW Parliament, 2 February 1998.

9. Lipski PS. "The Problem with Dementia Drivers". (Abstract presentation for the NSW Aged Care Assessment Team Conference, November 1998, Sydney.)

10. Lipski PS. "Driving and Dementia, and Nutrition in the Elderly". Invited speaker for The New Zealand Society for Geriatric Medicine Annual Scientific Meeting, Marlborough Sound, New Zealand, 19-20 November 1998.

11. Lipski PS. "Driving and Dementia - A Cause for Concern". Invited speaker for Physicians' Meeting. Tai Po Hospital, Hong Kong, 7 December 1999.

12. Lipski PS. "Undernutrition in the Elderly - A Cause for Concern". Invited speaker for Physicians' Meeting. Caritas Medical Centre, Hong Kong, 8 December 1999.

13. Lipski PS. "Undernutrition in the Elderly - A Cause for Concern". Invited speaker for Physicians' Meeting. Fung Yu King Hospital, Hong Kong, 9 December 1999.

14. Lipski PS. "Survey of General Practitioners' Attitudes to Older Drivers". Abstract. (Platform presentation for The Australian Society for Geriatric Medicine Annual Scientific Meeting, Cairns, July 2000.)

15. Lipski PS. "Unrecognised Dementia in Elderly Drivers". (Poster presentation for The Australian

Society for Geriatric Medicine Annual Scientific Meeting, Cairns, July 2000.)

16. Lipski PS. "Improving Food Delivery Services for Acute Hospital Geriatric Inpatients". A quality assurance project. (Poster presentation for The Australian Society for Geriatric Medicine Annual Scientific Meeting, Cairns, July 2000.

17. Lipski PS. "Survey of General Practitioners' Attitudes to Older Drivers". Abstract. (Platform presentation for the NSW Aged Care State Conference, 2002, University of NSW.)

18. Lipski PS. "Unrecognised Dementia in Older Drivers". (Poster presentation for The NSW State ACAT Conference, 2002, University of NSW.)

19. Lipski PS. "Improving Food Delivery Services for Acute Geriatric Inpatients". (Poster presentation for the NSW State ACAT Conference, 2002, University of NSW.)

20. Lipski PS. "The Impaired Older Driver". (Platform presentation for The Australian Association of Neurology Annual Scientific Meeting, Behavioural Neurology Symposium, Darling Harbour Convention Centre, May 2003.

21. Lipski PS. "The Impaired Older Driver". Presented to enquiry into road safety for older road users for the Victorian State Parliament Joint Standing Committee on Road Safety, 24 June 2003, NSW State Parliament.

22. Nutritional Care of the Housebound Elderly- Committee on Nutrition for Older Australians- Sydney University 4 Nov, 2005.

23. Lipski PS. Prospective audit of major drug reactions causing acute hospital admission of elderly patients. Australian Association of Gerontology Annual Scientific Meeting Gold Coast Queensland 2005.

24. Lipski PS. Geriatric Domiciliary Consultations – "A Dying Art". Australian Association of Gerontology Annual Scientific Meeting Gold Coast Queensland 2005.

25. New Zealand Dietetics Association Conference-Nutritional Care of the Housebound Elderly Christchurch NZ 3 Sept 2007.

26. The 2008 Gibson Oration: Malnutrition in the Elderly. Australian Association of Gerontology (Hunter Chapter). The annual Gibson Oration commemorates the work of the late R.M. (Dick) Gibson, pioneer of multidisciplinary geriatric care in the Hunter and founding member of the Australian Association of Gerontology.

## PUBLICATIONS

1. Holland RB, Levitt MW, Steffen CM, Lipski PS. "Intravenous cannulas, survey of their use in patients undergoing elective surgery". Medical Journal of Australia 1982; 2: 86-89.

2. Lipski PS, Kelly PJ, James OFW. "Bacterial Contamination of the Small Bowel in the Elderly. Is it necessarily pathological?" Age & Ageing 1992; 21: 5-12. (This paper is editorialised: "Clinical significance of bacterial overgrowth in elderly people" - Age and Ageing 1992; 21: 1-4.)

3. Lipski PS, Bennett MK, Kelly PJ, James OFW. "Ageing and Duodenal Morphometry". Journal of Clinical Pathology 1992; 95: 450-452.

4. Lipski PS, James OFW. "Small intestine" in: Grimley Evans J, Franklyn Williams T, EDS. Oxford Textbook of Geriatric Medicine. Oxford University Press 1992, pp 226-236.

5. Lipski PS. "Immobility: Causes and Consequences". Update in Geriatric Medicine, the Merck, Sharp & Dohme General Practitioner University Programme 1992.

6. Lipski PS. "Small Bowel Malabsorption in the Elderly". Update in Geriatric Medicine, the Merck, Sharp & Dohme General Practitioner University Programme 1992.

7. Lipski PS, Thomas JE, Mathers JC, Kelly PJ, Eastham OPW. "Blood, Ammonia and Helicobacter Pylori". Australian & New Zealand Journal of Medicine 1992; 22: 311.

8. Interview for Merck, Sharp & Dohme: Geriatric Medicine and the General Practitioner: Medical Education Newsletter MSD 1992, Vol2, No. 2.

9.Lipski PS, Torrance A, Kelly PJ, James OFW. "A Study of the Nature of Nutritional Deficits in Long Stay Geriatric Patients". Age and Ageing 1993; 22: 244-255.

10. Wallis JL, Lipski PS, Matthews JC, James OFW, Hirst BH. "Duodenal Brush Border Mucosal Glucose Transport and Hydrolase Activities in Ageing Man and the Effects of Small Intestinal Overgrowth". Digestive Diseases Sciences 1993; 38: 403-409.

11. Lipski PS. "Undernutrition in the Elderly - A Cause for Concern". Modern Medicine 1993; April pp 108-120.

12. Lipski PS. "Recent Advances in Geriatric Medicine. Continued Education and Current Perspectives". Fellowship Affairs, RACP. November 1993;23-26, 31-33.

13. Lipski PS, Death JW. "Risperidone in the Treatment of Agitated and Aggressive Patients with Dementia". Australian Journal on Ageing 1995; 13; No.4;151-154.

14. Lipski PS. "Hypertension in Elderly Hospital Inpatients". Pharmacy Bulletin, Central Coast Area Health Service. 1995. Vol 5. No.1.

15. Lipski PS. "The Consequences of Undernutrition in the Elderly". Proceedings of the Nutritional Society of Australia 1995; 19: 146-151.

16. Lipski PS. Editorial: "Optimum Care of the Elderly in an Acute General Hospital". Medical Journal of Australia 1996; 164: 5-6.

17. Lipski PS. "An Australian Nutrition Screening Initiative". Australasian Journal on Ageing 1996; Vol 15; No.1:14-15.

18. Lipski PS. "Driving and Dementia - A Cause for Concern". Medical Journal of Australia 1997; 167: 453-454.

19. Lipski PS. Position Statement No 6. Nutrition in the Elderly for the Australian Society of Geriatric

Medicine. Australian Journal on Ageing. 1997; Vol 16, No 4:174-178.

20. Lipski PS.  "Driving and Dementia".  Australian Dementia Care, 1999. April-May.

21. Lipski PS.  "Driving and Dementia.  Rights and safety".  National Health Care Journal 2000; May: 36-37.

22. Lipski PS, Hecker J.   "Dementia Behind the Wheel.  The debate:  Patients with signs of early dementia should retain a driving licence, provided they are subject to regular medical and driving assessments".  Australian Doctor; 2001: March 23; 62-64.

23. Lipski PS.   "Promoting the Quality Use of Medicines within Central Coast Health".  Drug Bulletin 2001; Vol.10; No. 1.

24. Lipski PS.  "A Survey of General Practitioners' Attitudes to Older Drivers on the NSW Central Coast". Australasian Journal on Ageing.  2002; June, Vol 21; No.2; 98-100.

25. Lipski PS.  "Improving Food Delivery Services for Acute Hospital Geriatric Inpatients.  A Quality Assurance Project".  Australasian Journal on Ageing. 2003; March. Vol 22; No.1; p44.

26. Lipski PS, Campbell P.  "Overlooking Orthostatic Hypotension in the Elderly".  Australasian Journal on Ageing. 2002; Dec, Vol 21; No.4; p213.

27. Bunt R, Lipski PS.  "Driving and Dementia.  A prospective audit of clients referred to an Aged Care

Assessment Team". Australasian Journal on Ageing 2003; December, Vol 22; No.4; p218.

28. Lipski PS. "Unrecognised Dementia in Older Drivers". Australasian Journal on Ageing 2003; June, Vol 22; No.2: p106.

29. Lipski PS. "The White Paper". A new direction for Geriatric Medical Services on the NSW Central Coast 2007.

30. Lipski PS. "Your Elderly Parents Failing Health. Is It Ageing Or A Treatable Condition?" GP Rounds. Central Coast News Letter. Brisbane Waters Private Hospital. July 2019.